Get Fit
Where
You Sit

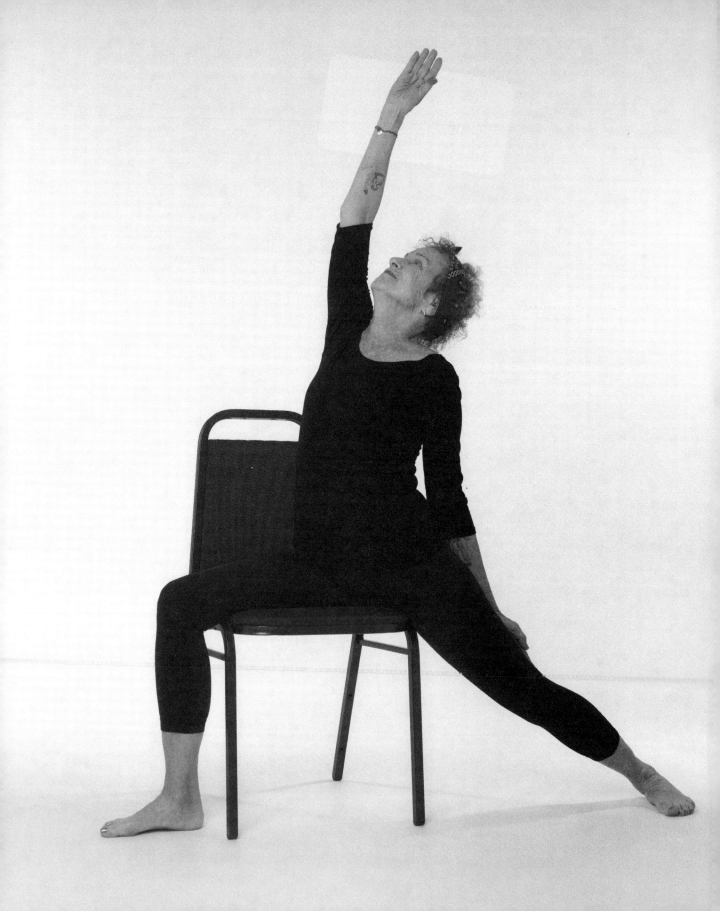

Get Fit Where You Sit

A GUIDE TO THE LAKSHMI VOELKER
CHAIR YOGA METHOD

Lakshmi Voelker
Liz Oppedijk

Foreword by Jivana Heyman
Photographs by Julie Frances Hopkins

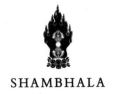

SHAMBHALA

Shambhala Publications, Inc.
2129 13th Street
Boulder, Colorado 80302
www.shambhala.com

The information in this book is not intended as a substitute for personalized medical advice. The reader should consult a physician before beginning this or any exercise program.

Cover Photo: Julie Frances Hopkins
Cover Art: ViSnezh/Shutterstock
Cover and interior design: Laura Shaw Design, Inc.

9 8 7 6 5 4 3 2

Printed in the United States of America

Shambhala Publications makes every effort to print on acid-free, recycled paper.
Shambhala Publications is distributed worldwide by Penguin Random House, Inc., and its subsidiaries.

Library of Congress Cataloging-in-Publication Data

Names: Voelker, Lakshmi, author. | Oppedijk, Liz, author.
Title: Get fit where you sit: a guide to the Lakshmi Voelker chair yoga method /
Lakshmi Voelker, Liz Oppedijk; Jivana Heyman (foreword writer) and
Julie Frances Hopkins (photographer).
Description: Boulder, Colorado: Shambhala, [2023] | Includes index.
Identifiers: LCCN 2022049897 | ISBN 9781611809251 (trade paperback)
Subjects: LCSH: Yoga. | Sitting position.
Classification: LCC B132.Y6 V634 2023 | DDC 204/.36—dc23/eng/20230126
LC record available at https://lccn.loc.gov/2022049897

To Anjali and Hymie Joseph, who set me on a lifelong path of deep inquiry, and to my beloved husband, Bruce.

—LAKSHMI

In memory of my dear husband Paul—my beloved buddy and biggest supporter, father to our wonderful children—with love and gratitude for all our blessings.

—LIZ

Being Present

Breathe, relax and feel;
take time to slow down
the pace of life. Watch the
rise and fall of moods, the
birth and death of dreams.
Feelings and sensations seem
so real, yet they shift like
changing clouds, and flow
with the high tide out to sea
again. Allow it all to be, no
need to grasp or push away.
Present with each moment,
the whole of you, body, mind
and soul, opens to receive.

—DANNA FAULDS,
*Go In and In: Poems from
the Heart of Yoga*[1]

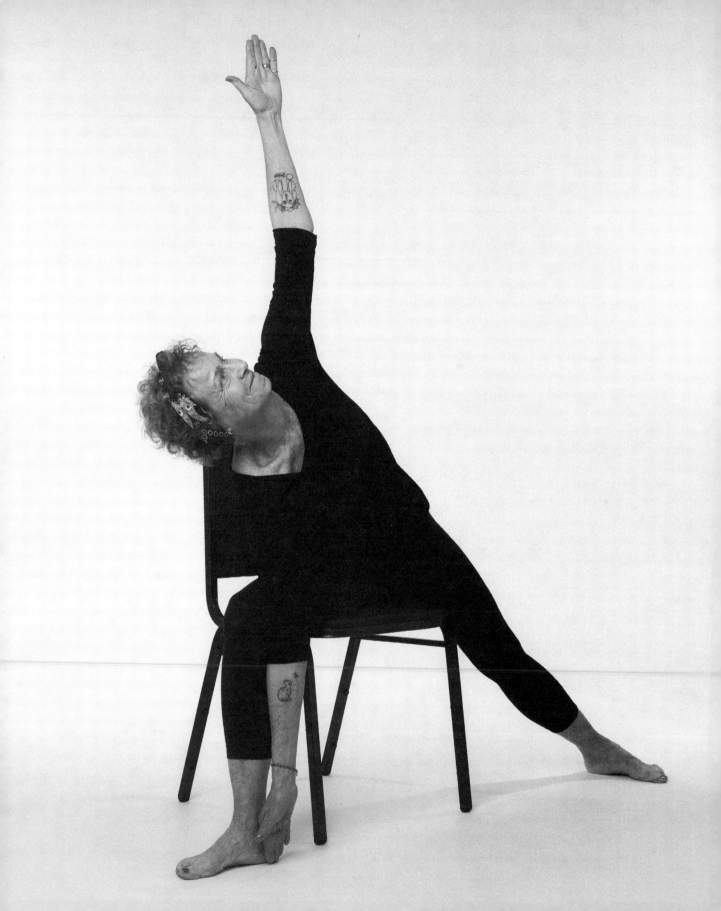

Contents

Foreword

THE OTHER DAY, I was looking through photos from one of our first Accessible Yoga Conferences, which took place in Santa Barbara, California, in 2016. The image that stood out most was a picture of Lakshmi Voelker teaching chair yoga with her arms stretched wide, energy flowing in her arms all the way out to her fingers, and her face gleaming with excitement. It's a remarkable photo because it truly captures her passion for yoga and how she is sharing it with the world.

Before that conference, I had heard of Lakshmi but never met her in person. She was already a legend in the world of accessible yoga, and it was exciting to meet and learn from her. Lakshmi showed us how practicing on a chair can transform an otherwise physically inaccessible practice into something truly available to an endless number of people who may otherwise never experience yoga.

What's most astounding about Lakshmi and her legacy as a yoga teacher is the dynamism and pure excitement that she transmits when she teaches. You get a sense of her energy in this book.

Liz Oppedijk arrived in my life at the perfect time. She helped to expand the work of Accessible Yoga, the nonprofit I founded, in the UK and Europe, and she kindly hosted me when I traveled to London. We taught together while I was there, which allowed me to see her in action. She offers a beautiful balance of humility and wisdom that shines through her teaching and also through these pages.

Over the years, I've come to see how it takes a powerful mind to take something complex and make it simple without losing its essence. The teachings in this book remind me of a line drawing by Pablo Picasso. With a single brushstroke he was able to capture the essence of his subject.

In the same way, these seemingly simple practices transmit the fullness of a complex and transformational tradition. This book helps to make the ancient, indigenous South Asian tradition of yoga accessible through creativity, exploration, and, above all, simplicity.

Not only will this book help you get fit where you sit, but it also extends the fullness of the yoga path to people of all ages and abilities. It even offers ways to practice when you don't have time to get on a yoga mat—at the office, sitting on an airplane, anywhere you find yourself. Held within these pages are simple techniques that offer transformation on many levels. It's a true gift for all of us.

—JIVANA HEYMAN

Acknowledgments

Lakshmi

First and foremost, I want to thank Liz Oppedijk, my coauthor. Liz, I don't know what I would have done without you. Your editorial expertise, your steadfast belief in the work and in me, and your collaborative spirit shine through every page of this book. I bow to you, my dharma sister.

My heart is full of gratitude to Shambhala Publications for taking on our book and birthing my and Liz's dream. Thank you to our incredible editor, Beth Frankl, and her team. You all believed in our book from the very beginning and gently but firmly worked to make it a reality. Hats off to assistant editors Peter Schumacher and KB Mello, designers Laura Shaw and Daniel Urban-Brown, publicist Katelin Ross, and marketer Johnnie Dina.

Thank you, Linda Sparrowe, for acting as our agent and being present every step of the way. You are a gifted editor and dedicated yogini. To Julie Hopkins, our keen-eyed photographer, model extraordinaire Brianna Pievac and her tricked-out wheelchair, and illustrator Michele Beckhardt-Lada. You all conspired to make our book extra special. And to Jivana Heyman for inviting our readers into the book by writing the perfect foreword. I am forever thankful for my daughter Heideli and my niece Donna who have been by my side for the three years it took us to birth the book. Daily texts, weekly phone calls, and visits supported my mission, which has been to bring yoga to everyone on this earth! And a loving shoutout to my dear friends Jenny Diaz, graphic designer extraordinaire whose work graces the pages of the book, and Linda Turner—you both mean the world to me!

A special thank-you to Candace Terry, who rolled out her towel alongside mine—almost fifty years ago—as we moved and stretched with Lilias and with Richard Hittleman on TV. By so selflessly sharing your own health challenges, you helped birth the very first Lakshmi Voelker Chair Yoga sequence. A deep bow to the five others who trusted me and allowed me to share LVCY in those early days: Catherine Holmes, Linda Dowd, Linda Malika, Jenny Diaz, and Darrell Franklin.

Lakshmi Voelker Chair Yoga would not exist without the many teachers whose wisdom and friendship guided me along the yogic path and continue to inform the LVCY method. I bow to Yoga Anand Ashram, Siddha Yoga, David North, who believed in me and encouraged me to "be a teacher of teachers," Thich Nhat Hanh, and Eckhart Tolle. To Kripalu Yoga Center, where I landed in the early 1970s and connected so deeply with the residents there, including Stephen Cope-Kaviraj, Deborah Orth-Rasmani, Kate Marchesiello, Rudy Peirce, and Chaula Hope Fisher—who supported my programs from the beginning—and Robert Quagliani, my driver, and Dave White, the security guard.

Hands to heart for all of my assistants, who lovingly, happily, and willingly served LVCY teacher trainings all over the country for decades. You were on target and on time every single time. Thom McGinley, Sandi Jacobs, Birgit Nagele, Grace Ho, Tracey Eccleston, Carmen Morente, and Brenda Yarnold were my very first assistants during the early 2000s. Followed by dozens of amazing ladies and gentlemen who gave of themselves selflessly year after year. A few of these assistants went on to become Master Trainers: Tracey Eccleston in Canada, Brenda Yarnold and Mandy Bush in the US, Claire Cunneen in Australia, and Liz Oppedijk and Stephanie Shanti Bosanko in the UK. I am grateful to all of you for tirelessly carrying on the tradition and making LVCY your own. I am also grateful to Howie Shareff for supporting LVCY for many years.

I will now finish by bowing to the Light in each and every one of my students who come back to class week after week, year after year, and decade after decade. I am eternally grateful to each and every one of you for believing in me and for eagerly embracing the miracle of Lakshmi Voelker Chair Yoga. I love you all!

Liz

I want to start by thanking Lakshmi. I am deeply honored and grateful to have worked with her, first as a student and then as a chair-yoga teacher trainer, and to offer my publishing knowledge as her coauthor. I feel grateful for discovering the wisdom and power of Lakshmi's chair-yoga approach and for the joy of making yoga accessible to anyone, especially those who are not able to practice yoga on a mat. Our special collaboration has produced this book and the wonderful opportunity to bring yoga and its therapeutic benefits to so many more people.

Adding to Lakshmi's words of gratitude, I would like to extend many thanks to all my amazing teachers and students, as well as to others who have helped us by sharing their wisdom at different stages of the book-creation process, including: Talya Baker, Jacky Bryant, Danna Fauld, Keeley Frampton, Dr. Bryony Hughes, Anne Luder, Heather Mason, Shweta Panchal, Jo Park, Kathy Ran, Matthew Taylor, Hayley Unwin, and Janice White.

My final thanks go to the memory of my precious husband, Paul, who passed away suddenly in the year of our book's birth, and to our beautiful children, Miriam and Ben. Their love, support, and steadfast belief in me give me the strength and courage every day to continue with my passion for offering accessible, healing yoga to those who need it.

We offer our book to those interested in chair yoga with positive intentions and having done our best to be honest and accurate. We trust that it will be received in this spirit.

Get Fit
Where
You Sit

Introduction

THE BIRTH OF CHAIR YOGA—LAKSHMI'S STORY

The year was 1967. I had just graduated from high school on Long Island, New York. With the whole summer spread out before me, I headed to the A&P grocery store with a friend, looking for something interesting to read. There by the cash register I noticed a collection of little Bantam books, two of which caught my attention: *The New Book of Yoga* by The Sivananda Yoga Centre and *Yoga U.S.A.: The Unique Exercise System 10 Million Americans Believe In* by Richard Hittleman, the star of the *Yoga for Health* program on TV. My curiosity piqued, I snapped them up right away and headed home.

I settled in on my couch to read. My friend was more interested in watching TV. Flipping through the channels, she found a yoga class with Richard Hittleman! Another channel featured Lilias Folan. Although all of this was new to me on one level, it felt oh so familiar as well. Nothing about it felt strange or foreign. I was "at home" with this new knowledge.

I spread out a bath towel on the floor and began practicing yoga in my Levi 501 jeans and my favorite madras blouse. This became a daily event for me—sometimes moving along with Richard and his "yoginis," other times breathing and stretching with Lilias. I was in love with it all.

Two years later, my friend Candace and I signed up for weekly yoga classes offered at our old high school as part of its adult education program. We arrived in our Levis and dangling silver bracelets, spread out our bath towels on the gym floor, and waited for the teacher to arrive. After a few moments, Anjali Joseph and her husband, Hymie, walked into the room and we began to practice. By the end of class, they had both taken up residence in our hearts. They became my first true teachers.

Fast-forward a few years: I joined Anjali and Hymie and others, and together we founded the Yoga Anand Ashram in downtown Amityville, New York—my hometown; the Santosha Vegetarian Dining restaurant soon followed downstairs. It was at the ashram that my studies began to deepen. I immersed myself in asana practice, yoga philosophy, women's studies, Indian cooking, and organic gardening. Yoga coursed through my veins.

At the same time, I threw myself completely into meditation. Fascinated by Transcendental Meditation (TM), Candace and I took the course and received our mantra. Bill, the TM governor, who lovingly prepared mung bean dahl and rice with loads of ghee on top, taught me the power of listening and the beauty of silence.

During this time, Siddha Yoga also entered my life. Daylong, weekend, and weeklong retreats opened me to my higher self, and knowledge and learning began to flow to and from me. I received *shaktipat* (the transmission of wisdom) from the teachers there and, in the tradition of Siddha Yoga, I was given my spiritual Sanskrit name, Mahalakshmi. I continued to grow and glow, and yet I had a feeling that something bigger was out there for me. I just didn't know what yet.

Unfortunately, all that sitting—hours, even days at a time—was hard on my body. A fellow meditator suggested I try Kripalu Center for Yoga and Health, not that far away in Lenox, Massachusetts. The moment I turned onto South Drive, with Lake Mahkeenac and Kripalu on my left and the forest and apple groves on my right, I knew I was home. Truly home.

I took many programs there and, finally, in 1982 I became certified as a Kripalu yoga teacher. Over the next few years, I added two more Kripalu certifications—one as a Kripalu bodyworker and another as a Danskinetics teacher. Although I learned from the senior teachers at Kripalu, my true teachers were the other students, all residents at the center like I was, who became, and remain, my brothers and sisters to this day.

I continued to teach mat yoga classes the way I had been taught, paying attention to alignment, moving from pose to pose on the wave of the breath. Standing, sitting, twisting, turning, forward and back, upside down and right side up.

And then one day in 1982, I got a phone call from Candace. Crying over the phone, she managed between sobs to let me know that her yoga days were over. She had been diagnosed with rheumatoid arthritis and the flare-ups were so intense she could no longer bend down to tie her shoes, zip up her jeans, or even drive a car. Yoga on the mat was out of the question.

I refused to believe that my dear friend could no longer benefit from yoga, that the gifts of yoga could be confined to only those who were already physically fit. I was determined to figure out a way to change up the practice. I thought and I thought and I thought. Alas, by the time the sun set I was no closer to a solution.

Discouraged, I turned my attention to my cat, Riddha Cat, who had leaped onto the coffee table in front of my chair and begun to meow. I extended my legs in front of me and hinged forward to see what the problem was. She jumped down to the floor and scurried under the table. I lowered my legs, flexed my feet, and began to rub her with my toes and the balls of my feet, lengthening my back as I did so. She then jumped back on the coffee table, so I drew my legs back toward the chair and moved toward the edge so I could talk to her.

I continued to follow Riddha Cat—she thought it was a great game. She moved over to a table on my right. In order to see where she went, I instinctively moved my right hand to the seat of the chair near my right hip and twisted my torso to the right so I could reach my left arm out to pet her. She loved it! But not content to stay in one place, she moved behind the chair (of course she did!) and I had to move into another level of flexibility to reach her. As I untwisted myself and came back to face the coffee table, I suddenly realized that, thanks to Riddha Cat, I had just created a whole yoga sequence—without ever leaving my chair! I had gone from a Forward Fold into Staff Pose and into a seated version of Mountain Pose, and then I had treated my spine to a marvelous seated twist.

I twisted to the other side to even things out. Then I drew stick figures on chairs and wrote simple instructions—and experimented with a few more poses. A day later, I gave it to Candace, who practiced the entire sequence every day for months. When she felt ready, she returned to class, bringing her chair with her. We both were amazed at the difference a simple chair could make, and yet for some reason, I didn't fully embrace these "chair-asanas" for a few more years.

Not long after that, I left Long Island for Desert Hot Springs in California, moved into a small trailer with a friend, did a stint as a store designer for JCPenney, taught a little more yoga, and felt like my life was finally coming together.

The late '80s and into the '90s saw more exploration that included learning from Deepak Chopra (a prominent Indian-American author known as an advocate of integrative medicine and self-transformation) and being in the presence of Thich Nhat Hạnh (Vietnamese Buddhist monk known worldwide as a spiritual leader, author, poet, teacher, and peace activist) and Eckhart Tolle (German-born spiritual teacher and author). I learned what it meant to be in the present moment through their books, videos, talks, and retreats—to be "in the now" was truly life changing for me. By 1999 I felt that chair yoga was ready for prime time, so I created an audio cassette entitled *The Sitting Mountain Series*.

From Desert Hot Springs I journeyed to Rancho Mirage, where I became the only yoga teacher in the desert. I was in demand. I quit my day job to begin teaching anywhere that would have me—country clubs, libraries, retirement homes, assisted living centers—and privately for the "rich and famous."

During that time, I met Maria Greenwald, MD, a rheumatology specialist with many decades of medical experience and a graduate of Yale Medical School, based in Palm Desert, who saw the value of chair yoga right away, and I began to sell my chair-yoga cassettes to her patients. Soon I was teaching chair yoga in the waiting room of her office. I played soft music, we meditated, and we did yoga on chairs. Patients joined in as they entered and stayed until their names were called for their appointments. Everyone loved it—including me. And I realized that I had found what had been missing all along—*the opportunity to bring all of yoga to anyone willing to give it a try, no matter what their level of mobility or flexibility.*

I could no longer ignore how stressful "conventional" yoga had become for so many who could and would benefit from its gifts: those who struggled to get up and down from the floor; those whose limited mobility caused them undue stress; those with large bodies who didn't feel safe or welcome. Let's face it: those not rich enough, thin enough, or bendy enough to fit into what had become our yoga "culture." My dharma, my raison d'être, became bringing the true teachings of yoga—including asana, pranayama, and meditation—into the lives of as many people as I could. I welcomed people with missing limbs, arthritis, chronic obstructive pulmonary disease (COPD), osteoporosis, heart disease, diabetes, multiple sclerosis (MS), dementia, cerebral palsy, and anyone else who felt "othered" or ignored. We practiced yoga on our chairs, sometimes using two chairs each to enrich the practice, and added light weights, blocks, bolsters, or straps—whenever those enhancements made sense. We chanted, we breathed, we moved, and we danced from our seats, supporting one another and embracing the beauty of our bodies and ourselves.

And we haven't stopped in more than fifty years!

In the decades since we started, the acceptance of yoga as a body-mind practice that can positively affect health and wellness has grown. The Lakshmi Voelker Method, in particular, is known as one of the most effective approaches to adapting yoga. Today, more than 2,500 teachers (and growing!) have gone through our training—60 to 65 percent of whom are not yoga teachers but rather a mix of health-care professionals, fitness professionals, dance teachers, educators, caregivers, therapists, and others—which allows yoga to expand exponentially and become accessible to a much broader population who might not otherwise reap its benefits. Every single one has added their own personal style to the practice and introduced it worldwide to an even more diverse population.

Sharing the Joy: Liz's Story

What I know firsthand is that anybody can do yoga, and it's never too late to start. I discovered yoga in my fifties following serious illness and injury, which ultimately left me with fragile bones. As a lifelong runner with a habit of falling, I needed to do something to improve my balance and flexibility. A friend suggested yoga, and to my amazement, it helped straightaway. When I next took a tumble, I fell "light"—no injuries. The second time I fell, I was running on the Champs-Élysées in Paris, when I suddenly tripped and slid across the pavement. No detectable damage (except to my ego); I was just sore around my abdomen. "That's your core," my yoga teacher explained. I had developed strength—doing yoga! I was hooked.

Three or four years after my graceful fall, my yoga teacher Kathy Ran opened a new studio, which attracted a clientele with relatively high levels of physical fitness. Kathy also wanted to help others do yoga, and she asked me to help her create a nonprofit. With my experience in community development and a master's degree in voluntary sector management, I thought it was a great idea, but I wanted to know more about yoga and why it works. So, I signed up for Kathy's 200-hour yoga teacher training. The learning, I soon discovered, was not just an intellectual exercise but an all-encompassing exploration of body, mind, and spirit—yoga truly delivering on the promises of its name.

When I finished the training, I had no real intention of teaching. But a friend begged me to teach the staff and parents at her kids' nursery, whose yoga teacher had just left. It was only a five-minute walk from my house: How could I refuse? I was struck by how stiff the staff were—young women in their twenties and thirties who had trouble getting up and down from the floor. Just as in my case, yoga helped them straightaway. They loved the increased physical flexibility, but they also craved (and raved about) feeling more relaxed. I started to think, "Isn't it great, what yoga can do for caregivers?"

Around this time, through my community work, I took part in a social action project in a local nursing home, where I observed the staff as they worked, and I wondered whether they would also benefit from yoga. And what about the residents? Clearly they wouldn't be able to do yoga on a mat. However, I remembered hearing about Lakshmi Voelker, a chair yoga specialist in America, so I emailed the trainer who had mentioned her, and she wrote back, "Lakshmi offers the BEST chair-yoga training around!"

The only challenge was that Lakshmi lives in California and I live in England. But as luck would have it, Lakshmi was already offering her training online—over a decade before the COVID-19 pandemic made Zoom a household word—so I signed up immediately. Then what could have been a disaster struck. While coming up from Toe Stand in a hot yoga class, I tore the meniscus in my right knee. Yet instead of feeling frustrated and irritated with the forced restrictions to my mobility, I felt my world actually expanding. Chair yoga, as I was learning it from Lakshmi, allowed me to adapt poses safely and effectively so I could carry on without missing a beat. I was hooked again—this time on the chair.

With my chair-yoga teacher training completed in 2016, I was ready to teach the residents at the local nursing home in earnest—and to conduct a little research. I was already convinced that yoga could be a wonderful activity to bring into nursing homes. I was particularly keen on seeing if it would help reduce the risk of falls for residents—a common occurrence among older people—and maybe bring some relief from depression and anxiety. After two months of teaching chair yoga twice a week, the feedback from both residents and staff was highly positive.

At the same time, I was asked to set up a new weekly chair-yoga class at the local YMCA for those with Parkinson's disease and multiple sclerosis. From its inception in 2016, and continuing online since 2020, this class has developed into a very special community. Those who attend have or are recovering from all sorts of physical conditions—stroke, cancer, arthritis, and diabetes, as well as Parkinson's and MS—and many come with partners, relatives, friends, or caregivers who may or may not have a few health challenges themselves. The Lakshmi Voelker Method allows me to guide those with and without health conditions, all in the same class! I love to adapt new things to the chair, and my students are willing participants, generously embracing my many experiments, including creating chair dance moves and—my newest passion—bringing qigong to the chair.

As I became more familiar with the yoga culture in the UK, I was surprised to discover how many people were put off from even trying yoga. "I'm not flexible enough." "I'm too old to do yoga." "Isn't yoga just for bendy young women in Lycra?" I knew that yoga could be made accessible to anyone, and I made it my mission to find a way to make that happen. In 2017, Lakshmi connected me with Jivana Heyman, the founder of the charity Accessible Yoga and the author of *Accessible Yoga* and *Yoga Revolution*. I am honored to have sponsored Jivana's first Accessible Yoga (AY) training in the UK and to facilitate regularly on his online AY training, which attracts students worldwide.

With input from the University of Hertfordshire and support from a range of funders, I also continued my research into whether it was feasible to offer yoga in nursing-home settings. A six-month pilot project in five local nursing homes in 2017–2018 delivered a resounding yes. Just before the first COVID-19 pandemic lockdown in 2020, we were able to complete the data collection for a third project, a small cluster study, which has shown yoga's positive effects in improving mood, relaxation, and social interaction as well as decreasing anxiety and depression for nursing-home residents with and without a dementia diagnosis.

Until this point, I had been offering only group chair-yoga sessions in nursing homes. But as I walked through the corridors of each nursing home, I couldn't help but notice how many people remained alone in their rooms. Maybe it was out of choice, or because they were ill or recovering from a fall. Whatever the reason, I felt that these people also deserved yoga—to help them feel better physically and emotionally. In order to provide that service, I decided I needed to become a yoga therapist.

I started looking at yoga-therapy training courses and found the Minded Institute, run by a remarkable yoga therapist, Heather Mason. Its evidence-based approach and its focus on mental health appealed to me from the start. Not only did the training expand my knowledge about yoga, but it also deepened my understanding of myself. Case in point: early on, when we covered anxiety, I finally allowed myself to admit and accept that I suffer with anxiety, too. I now lecture on the Minded course, teaching accessible yoga and chair yoga as well as modules on Parkinson's and dementia.

In 2019 I attended a National Health Service (NHS)–sponsored training on frailty, which had recently been recognized as a long-term health condition. The trainer defined frailty as "reduced resilience and increased vulnerability such that the person is less able to cope with and recover from accidents, physical illness, or other stressful events." As I listened to him speak, I suddenly realized that he was talking about me! *I was frail.* The osteoporosis that I had developed had emptied out my bones; my surgeon said he had never seen someone who didn't come from a developing country with such "bad bone disease." I have been able to rebuild my bones to a degree and greatly reduce frailty in my body, and yoga has been a crucial part of this recovery. In yoga, though, it is not enough to learn lessons simply for oneself. As my practice and teaching of yoga have progressed, I have been driven to bring yoga to those who are the most frail and vulnerable. One of my dreams is to create a model for bringing yoga to every nursing home in the UK (and beyond), and my nonprofit social enterprise, Accessible Chair Yoga CIC, has been set up to further this aim.

I often come back to the start of my yoga journey, which I began in later life. I still remember my first yoga class—a lovely warming vinyasa flow with an inspiring teacher in a chilly church hall near where I live in England. I remember what it was like to have never done yoga before: feelings of anticipation, fear, hope. What will it be like? Will I be able to do it? Will it help me? Then the class began and amazing impressions unfolded. Curiosity sparked by unfamiliar yet intriguing movements. The most wonderful feeling of stretch. And finally relief as we all settled into the final yoga rest pose. After the class, I felt invigorated yet also much calmer and relaxed in body and mind. And as I explored yoga week by week, I started to feel what I realized was joy—something I had as a child that had gotten lost in a busy and demanding life. By practicing and teaching the most accessible yoga possible, I am able to share my joy as well as help others access their own feelings of joy.

How to Use This Book

Yoga is only yoga when it becomes personal, when you make it your own; otherwise it's just exercise. Yoga becomes therapeutic, and even transformational, when the poses, breathing techniques, and meditation practices morph and change to fit your unique body, mind, and heart, instead of forcing your body into a predetermined, narrow definition of what yoga should look like. Ideally what you learn on the chair can then inform and enrich your daily life.

Whether you are currently a practitioner or simply curious enough to explore how yoga would fit into your life, we trust that this book will be of service. The yoga we present is designed to encourage you to experience the joy in every pose; to celebrate your unique qualities; and to stretch your imagination and creativity, as well as your body and mind, in ways that feel just right for you. If you are a yoga teacher or yoga therapist already, we invite you to try the chair on for size and, with an open mind, experiment with the different "levels of flexibility" that we offer and see how longstanding familiar poses can adapt themselves almost seamlessly to a chair seat.

We've chosen forty poses to explore on the chair, organized in alphabetical order. For each one, we offer at least three different ways to experience it, depending on your level of flexibility; point out the benefits and precautions; and suggest ways to incorporate breathwork, meditation, and other yoga techniques. We show what the pose looks like on the mat and then how it translates to the chair. Tips on how to make the most of the Lakshmi Voelker Method are interspersed throughout. Although we offer several sequences in these pages, we encourage you to get creative, to infuse those sequences with your personality—anything you'd like to bring to your experience. Why not? It's an opportunity to expand your understanding of what yoga really is and embrace all it has to offer you.

Our aim is to show how anyone can practice yoga on a chair safely and effectively and still receive and absorb the true essence of this ancient practice. To that end, we offer the basic teachings of yoga and then invite you to adapt your practice in any way that captures that essence for you.

Our aim is that this book will be the catalyst that awakens your desire to explore deeper, because there is so much more: double-chair yoga, pair-chair yoga, weighted chair yoga, acupressure massage on a chair, dancing on a chair, reflexology on a chair, qigong on a chair . . . and we encourage you to get in touch with us if you want to go further.

Now it's time to get fit where you sit!

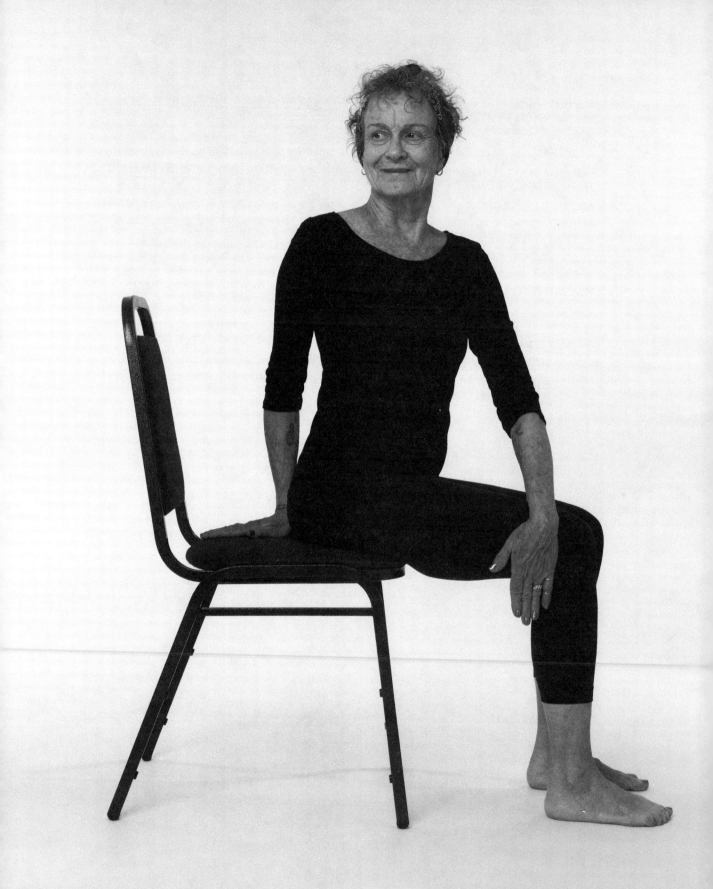

PART ONE

Take a Seat

1

Rise Up from the Slump

Posture (asana) is to be seated in a position which is firm but relaxed.

—SWAMI PRABHAVANANDA and CHRISTOPHER ISHERWOOD,
How to Know God: The Yoga Aphorisms of Patanjali

IN RECENT YEARS, all sorts of research studies and articles have warned of the perils of sitting too long. "Get up!" we're told. "Stand up! Sitting is bad for you." So why on earth do we recommend doing yoga on a chair?

Let's get the bad news out of the way first. Research does indeed show that prolonged sitting can be a problem, an issue further exacerbated by the 2019 coronavirus pandemic;[2] in fact, it can lead to "sitting disease," which can be as unhealthy as smoking cigarettes. When researchers talk about the symptoms of sitting disease, they often mention that a less active and more sedentary lifestyle leads to an increased risk of heart disease, high blood pressure, stroke, diabetes—and the list goes on. Poor posture is cited as a key contributor in back pain and work-related musculoskeletal issues,[3] and studies indicate that sitting and other sedentary behaviors reduce cerebral blood flow, which can lead to lower cognitive functioning[4] and an increase in mental health conditions, such as anxiety and depression.[5] And these risks are affecting the health of people all around the world.[6]

Sitting itself isn't necessarily the villain; it's the *way* and *duration* that we sit that can be problematic. Sitting disease symptoms often arise when we sit for extended periods of time—a kind of "slump-asana." When we slouch, our leg muscles slacken, which weakens the major muscles of the legs and buttocks and increases stress on the hip flexors. Over time, the hip flexors shorten, which heightens the risk of hip joint complications. Continuously sitting in this slumped posture puts pressure on the back; the head juts forward, which puts strain on the neck. This leads to uncomfortable muscle imbalances between the front and back body.

Over time, the load on the ligaments and intervertebral discs of the spine can contribute to chronic lower back and neck challenges, and restrictions in the chest can cause issues with the ribs and breathing. When we sit for long periods of time, especially in combination with a sedentary lifestyle, we may decondition any muscle group, including the major muscles of our legs and buttocks. This slumped body posture can also have a negative effect on our emotions and thoughts, with consequences for our mental and physical health.

We can avoid many of these issues by practicing *active sitting*, which helps us focus on postural alignment. Active sitting encourages us to sit with the bulk of our weight resting through the pelvis, particularly to the sit bones (the ischial tuberosities, or the lower part of the hip bone), so that the core structures of the abdomen, back, and hips can do most of the work against gravity to support an upright position and help maintain spinal stability. For active sitting, you'll often hear our chair-yoga teachers say, "Sit up on your chair—not down!" Our longtime chair-yoga student, Frances, is a testament to what we're talking about here. She is seventy-eight years old and has multiple sclerosis and has been taking weekly Lakshmi Voelker Method classes for several years. The combination of breath, movement, and relaxation techniques has definitely helped in her daily life. She was absolutely delighted when she could sit forward on the chair for an entire class—after only seven months of practice—without having to lean or collapse back. And, she says, things just keep getting better. A true tribute to the power of our approach to chair yoga to develop core strength and self-confidence!

Of course, sitting while doing yoga is hardly new. Its roots can be traced back to the early Upanishads, ancient Vedic texts written between 800 and 200 B.C.E., where techniques for controlling the breath and the mind first appeared. For millennia, yoga was primarily practiced while seated; every pose was in service to a stronger, suppler spine, one that would enable practitioners to sit for longer and longer periods of time—to achieve enlightenment. It seems that even the yogis of old knew it was hard to experience bliss if you're in excruciating pain.

Most styles of yoga still include breathing techniques (pranayama) and meditation, along with the physical postures (asanas). The difference is that Westerners need a lot more help than the ancient yogis did to sit cross-legged on the floor; many of us need something to "prop" us up—such as bolsters, cushions, blocks, and blankets—in order to gain some comfort. That's because most of us commute sitting in cars, on trains, or in buses; we work and play sitting on chairs and sofas—rarely in the most upright posture—all of which can cause tightness in the hips, weakness in the spinal muscles, and rounding in the back. These physical restrictions make sitting on the floor quite uncomfortable, if not pretty much impossible. On top of all that, many people admit that just the thought of having to get down onto the floor and up again—and the effort it takes—keeps them from enjoying and reaping the benefits of yoga's integration of body, mind, and spirit.

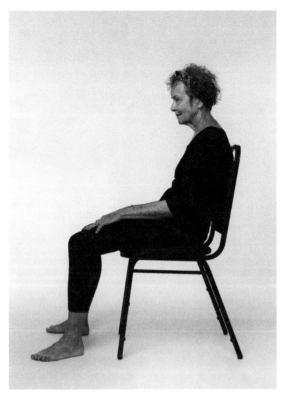 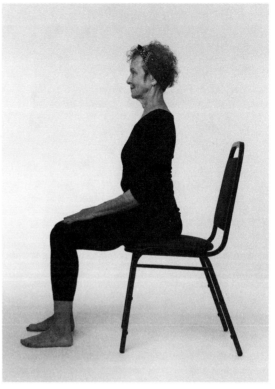

Slump-asana—a passive seated position

Sitting Mountain—an active seated position

Active Sitting

So what can we do to make sitting more comfortable and healthier? Begin by practicing active sitting on a chair, which is a great way to counter the negative impact of slump-asana. This technique works for anyone who has discomfort or pain in their hips, lower back, midback, upper back, shoulders, neck, or knees. This also includes anyone with limited mobility, injuries, or physical or psychological conditions that prevent them from sitting comfortably on the floor. Chair yoga provides a safer and more attainable alternative to traditional mat yoga.

Rising from slump-asana to Sitting Mountain (see page 42), a more upright posture, can help build strength in the legs and lower body, reduce rounding of the shoulders, improve breathing and posture, and lessen harmful loading on the spine (particularly vital for anyone who has bone loss or osteoporosis). Meditating in this posture on a chair—instead of on a cushion on the floor—can also help us find comfort and ease to quiet the mind, which can relieve anxiety without putting undue strain on the knees. Doing yoga on a chair allows us to adapt our practice to meet the needs of our body-mind on a given day, fostering strength, courage, and wisdom.

2

Who Benefits from Chair Yoga?

Yoga is for everyone.

—B. K. S. IYENGAR

WHO *DOES* BENEFIT from chair yoga? The short answer is: anyone! Just as with mat yoga, all aspects of yoga—conscious breathing, purposeful movement, mindful meditation—can be accessed and experienced when sitting on a chair.

Although the practice of yoga gets more popular every year, the health and healing opportunities it provides are not accessible to a large percentage of the population: people who either don't think their bodies fit the "yoga profile" or who are otherwise unable to participate in a fitness-focused mat yoga class. In a mat class, it can be too easy for the "ego" to override the intelligence of the body, causing people to either muscle into postures, hold them too long, or go further than their level of mobility, setting themselves up for injuries. Additionally, not being able to do the poses "as everyone else does" can be alienating—nobody likes feeling they aren't good enough. The chair yoga we describe throughout this book provides modifications that allow for people of all degrees of fitness to participate, creating a "level playing field" for everyone, which includes anyone:

- Living with a disability or with mobility challenges, including those who use wheelchairs or those with limited mobility due to conditions such as Parkinson's disease, multiple sclerosis, stroke, cancer, osteoporosis, scoliosis, arthritis, cerebral palsy, or muscular or skeletal imbalances. This also includes those who are unable to stand comfortably, who find balance difficult, or who may have lost their confidence after a fall or illness.

- With injuries or recovering from injuries, illness, or surgery. Chair yoga is used often in rehabilitation programs and, if appropriate, as a transition back to mat yoga and/or other sports and physical activities.

- Whose work requires frequent lifting, such as health-care workers, caregivers, and those in physically demanding professions (e.g., emergency services, retail, construction). It is particularly beneficial to facilitate a deeper stretch in the lower back and for lumbar-pelvic-hip flexibility.

- Who sits at a desk all day or travels often. It's ideal whenever getting on the floor is impractical.

- Facing psychological, emotional, or mental health challenges. It helps to find grounding (stability) and relief from stress through appropriate asanas, pranayama, and meditation.

- Who needs techniques to support mobility and independence as their body ages. It helps maintain flexibility, coordination, muscle strength, and bone mass.

- Who is pregnant, to promote a sense of calm and foster a positive attitude. It is particularly helpful in keeping the body in good physical shape during pregnancy and in preparing the body and mind for the birthing process.

- Who is in their childhood or teenage years. It's ideal to develop concentration, relieve stress, and encourage bonding with family and friends.

- Who lives or works in a place where movement is limited or restricted. This includes offices, nursing homes, hospitals, schools, prisons, and the like.

- Who cares for or serves others and needs a holistic health-care tool to ensure self-care for themselves.

- Who finds mat yoga intimidating or uncomfortable and wishes to practice in a compassionate and comfortable environment where every *body* can participate at their own level.

A Word about Sanskrit and Language

Yoga was first formulated in Sanskrit, an ancient language of India. To honor its long history and tradition, we use Sanskrit words throughout, as appropriate. To ensure that the content is accessible to all, we explain the yoga philosophy from which our approach to chair yoga is drawn and include a glossary at the back of the book. We invite you to come to the material with an open and curious mind: sometimes words—both familiar and unfamiliar—can offer an opening to healing by allowing us to think in new ways and helping us to break old habits that harm or no longer serve us.

Please note: Sanskrit words and spellings for asanas, pranayama, and yoga concepts are open to many interpretations. We researched numerous explanations through many books and sacred texts. Working with a diverse group of professionals, Lakshmi Voelker Chair Yoga teachers, and students brought us much to contemplate along this journey. Our use of Sanskrit for each asana, pranayama, and yoga concept is our understanding based on this research.

A Special Note for Teachers

Our approach to chair yoga draws its inspiration in part from Tirumalai Krishnamacharya, often referred to simply by his last name and known as "the father of modern yoga" for his influence on how postural yoga has developed in modern times. He wrote, "In recommending yoga practices, teachers should always consider an individual's particular circumstances. Just as other activities and practices must be adapted to the changes in one's life, such as aging, so too, yoga practices need to be adapted as the practitioner changes."[7] Using the chair yoga we describe throughout this book makes room for you to be as creative as you want in your practice and your teaching, which sets it apart from many styles of yoga that have strong ties to lineage and teach a fixed set of practices. This chair-yoga method provides you with the skills and confidence to create practices that are truly accessible to anyone and any *body* on any chair. You will be fully empowered to offer safe, effective, imaginative, fun, and inspiring practices for yourself as well as for whatever populations you serve.

The Lakshmi Voelker Method Mission Statement offers yoga professionals and those who want to share the Lakshmi Voelker Method with others the following intention:

- To bring yoga's integration of body, mind, and spirit to those unable to practice traditional mat yoga.

- To create an environment of safety by:

  » Instructing each student in ways to safely enter and exit each pose.
  » Teaching each student when and how to do a pose and when and how not to do a pose, given their body-mind challenge.
  » Having an expanded awareness that every *body* is different.
  » Teaching each class knowing that there will be varied levels of ability and expertise in each class.

- To observe and honor each student and their differences.

We trust that anyone interested in adapting yoga safely and effectively to the chair— whether you are a yoga teacher, yoga therapist, health-care professional, exercise or fitness specialist, caregiver, community worker, or someone who simply wants an accessible way of gaining yoga's benefits—will use this book as a guide, a resource, and an inspiration for practicing this method of chair yoga or becoming trained to teach it.

As we always say, "If you're breathing, you can do yoga." So find a chair, take a seat, and get fit where you sit!

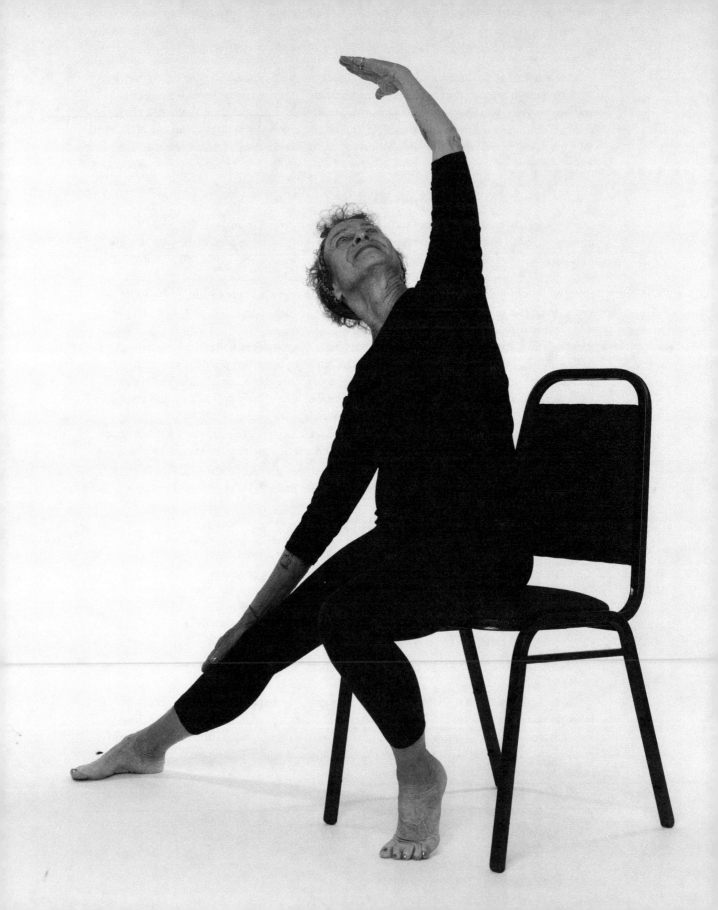

PART TWO

The Lakshmi Voelker Method

3

Roots, Principles, and Philosophy

In the practice of yoga, one can emphasize the body, the mind,
or the self and hence the effort can never be fruitless.

—KRISHNAMACHARYA

THERE ARE PLENTY of ways to use chairs in a yoga class to give students extra support when they need it—most often that means placing a chair next to a mat as a way to get down to the floor and up again, or as a prop to hold on to during balancing poses or standing poses. In other words, using a chair can help students keep up with others who are more flexible, stronger, more able-bodied, or more fit than they are. The problem with that premise, of course, is that there is no "more" in yoga, no comparisons to make, no place to get to. Every person's practice is unique to them.

Chair yoga can be a complete practice in itself, one in which the student never leaves their chair. While most chair yoga is posture-based, this book's approach is grounded in all eight limbs of the ancient practice in an empowering, enlightening, and joyful way. Along with our asana and pranayama sequences, a typical session might touch upon how we treat one another; how we honor ourselves; how we listen to and connect with our bodies; and how we use conscious breathing and meditation to relax the body, clear the mind, and open the heart to goodness and compassion.

In the following pages, we'll explore our teaching philosophy and how these key influences and philosophical underpinnings provide an effective way of meeting the needs of our teachers and students.

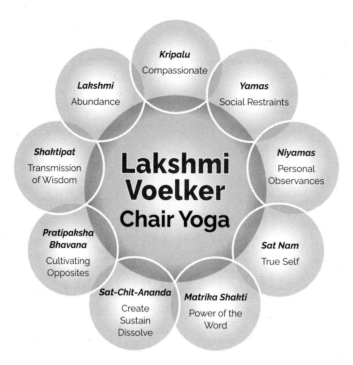

The diagram shows "Lakshmi Voelker Chair Yoga" at the center, surrounded by:
- **Kripalu** — Compassionate
- **Yamas** — Social Restraints
- **Niyamas** — Personal Observances
- **Sat Nam** — True Self
- **Matrika Shakti** — Power of the Word
- **Sat-Chit-Ananda** — Create Sustain Dissolve
- **Pratipaksha Bhavana** — Cultivating Opposites
- **Shaktipat** — Transmission of Wisdom
- **Lakshmi** — Abundance

Compassionate (*Kripalu*)

Kripalu (Sanskrit for "compassionate")—both the place and the style—has played a central role in the development of the Lakshmi Voelker Method. Founded in the 1970s, Kripalu yoga is a challenging approach that emphasizes meditation and breathwork, encouraging inward focus and spiritual harmony. Practicing Kripalu yoga can initiate a gradual process of physical healing, psychological growth, and spiritual awakening. Today the name Kripalu also refers to the Kripalu Center for Yoga and Health, located in the beautiful Berkshires of western Massachusetts; it is the largest yoga-based retreat center in North America.

Kripalu's Meditation in Motion, also known as Riding the Wave of Alignment, is an integral part of our chair-yoga approach, which is at its heart infused with compassion, empathy, care, and loving-kindness, qualities that resonate and speak to the needs of both teachers and students. Riding the Wave of Alignment is a three-stage methodology that we've adapted to our chair-yoga practice.[8]

Please note that these stages are not necessarily linear. Once you are familiar with yoga, you can move around the three stages in any order you desire.

STAGE ONE: LEARNING

- The focus is on anatomical safety and correct alignment on the chair—learning how to breathe into each asana, how to listen to your body, and how to do only what feels good.

- Your ego and will (desire)—the power of choosing your actions—are in ascendance.

- This stage is about asana and pranayama—body and breath awareness.

STAGE TWO: BALANCE

- The focus is on moving within and attuning to internal sensations with compassion and awareness—bringing the right and left hemispheres of your brain into balance and into a healthy partnership with your body.

- Your will (desire) combines with elements of surrender—letting go.

- This stage is about indulging your body-mind in each asana with the aid of deep, focused pranayama—holding the posture assisted by your breath.

STAGE THREE: SPONTANEOUS MOVEMENT

- This is where you feel an intuitive guidance moving through you when you move from one position (asana) to another. You offer your body to your spirit, allowing prana (life-giving force) to be your guide and your controlling mind to release its duties as the authority.

- Relaxing your ego and qualities of surrender are in ascendance.

- This stage is about "meditation in motion," or free and natural posture flow—trusting yourself inside and out—and following your inner chair-yoga teacher!

Transmission of Wisdom (*Shaktipat*)

In some lineages, the senior yoga teacher—sometimes called a "guru"—is considered to be the chief proponent and fount of all important knowledge, the leader who decides how and to whom wisdom may be transmitted or handed down. This process of "handing down," where the guru transfers their wisdom when the student is deemed ready, is known in Sanskrit as *shaktipat*, which translates literally as "prostration of strength."

In our chair-yoga practice, we use the word *shaktipat* in a broader and more inclusive way. Our approach is filled with shaktipat: it is informed by the teachings, blessings, and wisdom passed down from many ancestors, masters, teachers, and gurus from the past and the present, such as Krishnamacharya, Swami Kripalu, and others who are quoted in this book. We consider this concept as a way for us to acknowledge and honor those we learn from, no matter who they are. The transmission of their knowledge is not contingent on the opinion of the teacher as to a student's readiness, nor does it always travel in the direction from teacher to student. As teachers, we are also always learning from our students. Everyone has access to these teachings: we can all receive—as well as give—shaktipat!

We interpret shaktipat as something personal and nonjudgmental; something that fosters self-discovery. The process of gaining and communicating teachings will be different for each person, depending on their own experience. Once these teachings are transmitted, they no longer belong to the teacher. As a student or teacher, once you absorb the Lakshmi Voelker Method, you are gifted with shaktipat. You are then empowered to use these teachings how you wish. And then you will pass them on to others in your own way (see "True Self (*Sat Nam*)," page 28). We encourage you to continue to seek out your own teachers, then take their teachings and knowledge and develop your own experiences and wisdom.

Patanjali's Eight Limbs of Yoga

Our approach to chair yoga is also steeped in yoga philosophy as it is presented by the great sage Patanjali. Who was Patanjali? Translated from the Sanskrit, *pat* can mean "to fall," and *anjali*, "divine offering," suggesting the gesture his mother, Gonika, was said to have made with her hands while praying for a baby. The myth of Patanjali is that the god Vishnu decided to let his grace fall upon this sweet woman and thus Patanjali was born.

Patanjali united many different ideas about yoga into his classic work *The Yoga Sutras of Patanjali*. These sutras, or "threads," are short aphorisms articulating yogic wisdom we can incorporate into our everyday lives. Ultimate happiness or yoga can be achieved by reading, studying, absorbing, and practicing each sutra. In particular, chapter 2 of the *Yoga Sutras* outlines eight principles, or "limbs," of yoga, also called the Ashtanga path, a well-known framework followed by ancient and modern yogis for a more conscious and peaceful life, one of connection and purpose.

This path includes: *yama* (restraint), *niyama* (observance), *asana* (seat or posture), *pranayama* (breathwork), *pratyahara* (turning inward), *dharana* (concentration), *dhyana* (meditation), and *samadhi* (absorption). Each of these limbs helps us shift from limited to expanded awareness. They are not sequential stages but independent entry points leading to an expanded sense of self; through interpretations, choices, and experiences, they remind us of our essential nature, which can be understood as who we are, independent of what we do. Let's review each of these principles.

YAMAS

Yamas, translated as "social restraints," are five precepts that give us guidelines for social behavior—how we act toward others.

1. *Ahimsa*: nonviolence
2. *Satya*: truthfulness
3. *Asteya*: nonstealing
4. *Brahmacharya*: moderation
5. *Aparigraha*: nonpossessiveness

NIYAMAS

Niyamas, translated as "personal observances," are five principles that offer us guidelines for personal behavior—how we act toward ourselves.

1. *Saucha*: purity
2. *Santosha*: contentment
3. *Tapas*: self-discipline
4. *Svadhyaya*: self-study
5. *Ishvara pranidhana*: surrender to a higher power

PUTTING THE YAMAS AND NIYAMAS INTO PRACTICE

Swami Kripalu said, "By firmly grasping the flower of a single virtue, a person can lift the entire garland of yama and niyama." How do we use the yamas and niyamas in our chair-yoga practice? Below we share important aspects of each one and offer suggestions on how to apply them when practicing yoga on the chair as well as in your daily life. (See also pages 32–33 for ideas on how to practice these limbs while meditating sitting on a chair.)

AHIMSA: Awareness and gentleness in action, thought, and speech

Practice: Using compassion, understanding, patience, self-love, and worthiness

For Teachers: Ahimsa reminds us to consider a gentler, more compassionate approach to ourselves, our students, and everyone around us. We do this by providing levels of flexibility, honoring each of our students exactly as they are in that moment, and creating a class that is safe for all.

SATYA: Truthfulness of speech, thought, and deeds

Practice: Honesty, owning our feelings, loving communication with ourselves and others, non-judgment, forgiveness, letting go of facades

For Teachers: Truthfulness applies to letting our own voice shine through as teachers, coming from an honest and open perspective without judgment. It invites our students to be honest with themselves and show up in ways that honor their bodies, their emotions, and their energy—in the moment.

ASTEYA: Not coveting, not acting out of jealousy

Practice: Using objects the right way, proper time management, cultivating a sense of completeness, self-sufficiency, letting go of cravings

For Teachers: Practicing asteya means more than not stealing physical items. As practitioners or teachers, we sometimes feel that our good health has been "stolen" due to illness or injury. The levels of flexibility in our chair-yoga approach help shift feelings of loss toward greater acceptance and gratitude for what we do have and what we can do.

BRAHMACHARYA: No overindulgence of mind, intellect, speech, or body; moderation on all levels concerning food, sex, and all aspects of daily life, including the environment

Practice: Not repressing but managing and balancing sensual cravings

For Teachers: Committing to brahmacharya on the chair means focusing our energy during practice so that we maintain constancy and moderation and encourage our students to do the same.

APARIGRAHA: Fulfilling needs rather than wants

Practice: Nonattachment to possessions and relationships; generosity

For Teachers: Aparigraha reminds us to not be attached to a one-shape-fits-all approach to a pose. It also helps us encourage students not to be attached to the way someone else does a pose, which could result in either shame ("I'm doing it wrong!") or injury ("My pose has to look a certain way regardless of how it feels.").

SAUCHA: Purity of body, cleanliness, good health habits

Practice: Evenness of mind, thought, speech, and perception

For Teachers: When we use saucha as a centering meditation in class, we can offer a way for students to cleanse their minds and hearts of self-doubt or judgments.

SANTOSHA: Acceptance of what is; making the best of everything

Practice: Gratitude and joyfulness; remaining calm with success or failure; a state of mind that does not depend on any external status

For Teachers: Offering santosha and gratitude together as a centering meditation can encourage our students to be content with and grateful for what their bodies can do and let go of expectations around what their bodies should be able to do.

TAPAS: The willingness and discipline to do what is necessary to reach a goal; the discipline to choose freedom and joy, even when life is demanding, restrictive, or burdensome

Practice: Determination to pursue daily practices; enthusiasm for a spiritual path; joyfulness with outer discipline that will lead to inner discipline

For Teachers: Tapas cultivates a sense of self-discipline, passion, and courage to burn away impurities—physically, mentally, and emotionally. It is what gives us the desire and resolve to show up fully for our students and ourselves, and it gives us the willpower we need to commit to the practice in our daily lives.

SVADHYAYA: Expanding knowledge through reading, pondering on, and striving to understand new learning; engaging in observation of the self in relation to all of life as a means of personal growth

Practice: Studying yogic and other texts, reflection, and meditation; wanting to seek knowledge and truth; committing to lifelong learning; bringing a sense of self and self-awareness into our practice and into our everyday lives

For Teachers: Svadhyaya allows us to stay curious, be open to always learning about ourselves through self-study, movement, and breath. It helps us stay open to learning from our teachers as well as from our students. Svadhyaya, which keeps us grounded in the present, is the essence of chair yoga and meditation. It helps us as teachers and as practitioners pay attention to each body part and to the whole asana.

ISHVARA PRANIDHANA: Setting appropriate goals and directions in life and surrendering accomplishments and desires of the ego to a higher power, be it the self, the universe, or a deity

Practice: Dedication, sincerity, humility, and patience to transcend the ego, which is so resistant to surrender

For Teachers: Ishvara pranidhana means "surrender to the Divine." It reminds us to stay humble, to remember that yoga is not about us. We serve as guides for the students we teach, passing on the gifts we have received from others before us—and from the practice itself. We are vessels of the Divine; and when we give ourselves up to the process, we trust the divine knowledge and wisdom to lead us through the best possible experience.

ASANA

Asana is the physical posture or pose, the full physical representation of the body-mind connection. The postures are designed to create balance, strength, flexibility, and coordination. As we practice asanas, we begin to bring yoga into our daily life. Through the practice of asanas, yoga truly begins to be lived through our whole body-mind.

PRANAYAMA

Pranayama is the science of breath. Combining *prana* (life-giving force) with *yama* (restraint) encourages conscious control of the breath, mastering the life energy. Another translation of *pranayama* combines *prana* as "breath" with *ayama*, which means "extension" and can be understood as breathing techniques that allow us to intentionally control and extend the breath. At a cosmic level, it is the vital energy that vibrates through nature and the universe. At an individual level, pranayama is available to everyone: as we control and master our breath, we extend and master our lives.

PRATYAHARA

Pratyahara is the withdrawal of our senses from the world. We are then able to hear our inner voice more clearly. It is the process of directing the senses inward to become aware of the subtle elements of sound, touch, sight, taste, and smell. While both asana and pranayama are mindful activities, it is here where we begin intentionally to train our mindfulness "muscle," bringing our awareness more consciously into the present moment.

DHARANA

Dharana is the concentration or gathering of the mind—to hold, to carry, to maintain and resolve. It is the mastery of attention and intention. Whatever we place our attention on grows. Dharana invites us to develop an understanding of and be aware of our intentions.

DHYANA

Dhyana is meditation—it is the development of awareness. Through practicing meditation and Yoga Nidra ("yogic sleep," a form of guided meditation or deep effortless relaxation), we can cultivate this state of ever-present witnessing awareness directly.

SAMADHI

Samadhi is the state of being settled in pure, unbounded awareness, sometimes referred to as a state of complete self-absorption, enlightenment, or bliss. Combining our consciousness with meditation to reach a state of clarity, we tap into the core of who we are, our essential nature.

The eight limbs of Patanjali yoga, particularly the yamas and niyamas, provide the foundation upon which our chair-yoga method was created and built. We encourage teachers and practitioners to explore these guidelines for living with meaning, purpose, and wellness and discover for themselves how these concepts may relate to their own lives.

True Self (*Sat Nam*)

Sat nam is a Sanskrit word that is often used as a chant or mantra (see chapter 11). In our chair-yoga practice, sat nam is a key element—for both teachers and practitioners—in forming our own individual identity; it's part of our own personal journey of growth and development. *Sat* means "truth," and *nam* means "name"; together, *sat nam* translates as your "true name" or "true identity." When used as a greeting, *sat nam* means "I see your true nature" or "I recognize the divinity within you."

As a teacher, you adapt poses in levels of flexibility based on your experience of them on the mat (as available), before you adapt the pose on the chair, starting with your fullest expression and working down to the simplest expression (see chapter 7). Endless stores of creativity become available to you in guiding your students, which help you develop and bring your own sat nam—your own unique style, voice, interests, and authentic self—to the chair. You use your sat nam to teach *your* way, not *our* way.

As a practitioner, you can use your sat nam to adapt poses for yourself, which is empowering. You can take responsibility for your own yoga and what works best in your own body, whether you're doing chair yoga on your own or in a class. When you start to explore levels of flexibility in a pose, experimenting with different options that benefit your body-mind, you have truly embarked on your own personal yoga journey.

We use sat nam in our practice and our teaching to remind ourselves and our students of who we truly are. Our unique personality comes forth, and we practice and teach chair yoga from that grounded, assured place within. As Mahatma Gandhi said, "If you want to change the world, start with yourself."

The Power of the Word (*Matrika Shakti*)

Matrika shakti is a concept that appears in the Indian text *Shiva Sutras. Matrika* represents the vibration of sound that shapes letters, words, and thoughts; *shakti* means "power." Together *matrika shakti* can be translated as "the power of the word." It refers to the energy connected to the letters in the alphabet; the words in a sentence; the sound vibrations that create thoughts, feelings, and speech—illustrating and acknowledging the tremendous power of language. How we use words is important. For example, if we tell a child who seems awkward or trips or falls often that they are so clumsy that they could stumble over a thread on the floor, then there is a good chance that this child will not have the confidence to become a ballet dancer!

In our approach to chair yoga, we take care to use our language consciously and deliberately, preferring, for example, to use the word *challenge* instead of *pain, illness, disease,* or *ailment.* Using a neutral word like *challenge* removes any negative connotations or energy and focuses on kindness. Instead of saying "I have a bad back or a bad knee," we might say, "Today, my back is giving me a challenge." Saying it this way removes judgment and reminds us that we have no "bad" body parts, that what's happening is not permanent, and that we can reassure our back or knee that we aren't imposing any time limit for healing. Using *challenge* allows the body part to heal tomorrow, next week, or perhaps next year. If the challenge is permanent—a disability that won't physically heal—the "healing" may be in learning a new way to work with it.

As teachers, our language determines the effectiveness of our teaching. It's important to pay attention to how we phrase things—and notice how our students speak about themselves and their bodies. When we encourage students not to identify with their challenges, their consciousness rises to a more loving body-mind connection. Further, the meaning of words and how people receive them can change, so it is essential to revisit the language we use from time to time. In this way, our communication can remain as effective as possible.

Following the principles of matrika shakti in both spoken and unspoken communication allows each student to understand and feel fully included. For example, not everyone is familiar with Sanskrit; some students may find it confusing, excluding, and even off-putting when teachers use it during class. Instead of automatically using Sanskrit, teachers may ask students what they prefer and then slowly introduce new yoga words and concepts when that feels appropriate and inclusive. In our chair-yoga approach, we practice matrika shakti by offering multiple levels of flexibility (see page 81)—using verbal instructions (spoken language) and physical demonstrations (body language)—to encourage every practitioner to find an accessible variation of each yoga technique that is appropriate for them on that day. This ensures that every practitioner is able to participate; no one feels left out. In addition, learning new words and stimulating new movements taps into the brain's "plasticity"—its ability to change and form new neural connections—contributing to our overall health and wellness as well as our capacity to recover from illness or injury.

Matrika shakti is the powerful energy vibration of the sounds that make up our internal truth. It is so powerful it can change your life in a moment. Using the energy within matrika shakti, you can create bliss or wreak havoc with the "power of the word." "Sticks and stones may break my bones, but words will never hurt me"—does this childhood rhyme ring a bell for you? It needs to be: "Sticks and stones may break my bones, but words can hurt forever." It actually might be easier to recover from a broken bone than to recover from a hurtful word! It's important to become acutely aware of the words you speak on a day-to-day basis. Notice the impact you have when you're not being very nice and you say mean things to someone versus the impact you have when you *are* being kind and you say loving things to someone. The unruliness of the mind is simply the play of matrika, often outside our conscious awareness. You can become your own internal observer (the witness) who watches the nonstop activity of matrika shakti, the power of the word.

Matrika shakti reminds us to take note of these words written by Andy Rooney, an American radio and television writer: "Always keep your words soft and sweet, just in case you have to eat them."

Create-Sustain-Dissolve (*Sat-Chit-Ananda*)

Sat-chit-ananda is a Sanskrit word composed of three smaller words—*sat*, meaning "truth"; *chit*, meaning "consciousness"; and *ananda*, meaning "bliss." It can be translated overall as "truth, consciousness, bliss" or more actively as "create, sustain, dissolve." In the *Taittiriya Upanishad*, an ancient yoga text, it declares of human beings, "In bliss they were conceived, in bliss they live, to bliss they will return."

The cycle of life: Everything in life can be seen as sat-chit-ananda. Something is created (conceived), then sustained (lived), and eventually dissolved (returned), affording the opportunity to create (conceive) again. For instance, you plant an acorn; it grows into a tree, which perhaps gets hit by lightning and burns or simply dies. Meanwhile, an acorn from that tree starts the cycle again. Sat-chit-ananda shows up in our chair-yoga practice: we create a pose in our body-mind, we sustain the pose with the breath, and then we dissolve the pose, returning to Sitting Mountain and then on to another asana or pranayama.

Everything is part of a process that begins, continues, ends, and starts all over again—in our relationships, our work, our education, our health . . . The cycle of life goes on. When we view life as this continuous cycle, we gain a framework that supports us and provides perspective in dealing with change—both for changes we seek and those we don't.

SAT-CHIT-ANANDA AND THE POWER OF THREE

Sat-chit-ananda is a wonderful illustration of the power of three. Throughout history, the number three has had unique significance in different cultures. For instance, the ancient Greeks considered three to be a "perfect" number, a symbol of harmony, wisdom, and understanding. In addition to the meanings described above, we love the comparison of sat-chit-ananda to an apple on an apple tree. The apple blossom sprouting on the tree is sat, the fruit as it grows is chit, and the fully matured and ripened apple that is ready to fall or be plucked from the tree is ananda. In yoga, the cycle of three can be seen and integrated in many further ways:

- Three sounds in OM, the universal sound, pronounced *ah-oh-umm*: *ah* is create, *oh* is sustain, *umm* is dissolve. (See page 204.)

- Three breaths in asana: The first breath nurtures and nourishes the body. The second breath clears the mind. The third breath lifts the body-mind to the spirit's height and joy.

- Three press points in the feet: The first is below the big toe in the ball of the foot. The second is below the little toe in the ball of the foot. The third is in the center of the heel. Lift your toes off the ground and anchor all three press points in your feet down onto the ground for active sitting on the chair. (See pages 42–43)

- Three steps to your fullest asana expression: Adapt. Activate. Achieve the benefits.

- Three affirmations at the end of a chair-yoga session: Bringing your palms together in Anjali Mudra at your heart center, raise your hands so the index fingertips touch your forehead for clear thoughts, then your lips for kind words, and then back to your heart for loving compassion.

- Three parts to a rich and full chair-yoga practice: conscious breathing, purposeful movement, mindful meditation.

Cultivating Opposites (*Pratipaksha Bhavana*)

Practicing the chair-yoga approach presented in this book helps fosters a positive attitude. One way we do that is by subscribing to *pratipaksha bhavana*, the yogic practice of shifting negative ways of thinking or acting by "cultivating the opposite." According to Patanjali in his *Yoga Sutras* (2:33–34), "When disturbed by negative thoughts, opposite [positive] ones should be thought of. This is pratipaksha bhavana." We can practice pratipaksha bhavana by taking an active, conscious, and mindful approach to changing any destructive, negative, or untrue thoughts or actions we may have, and this helps us to embrace the yamas and niyamas.

How do we change negative ways of thinking? One way is by being aware of our words (*matrika shakti*) and choosing positive, kind, and nonharmful words when speaking to others and to ourselves (*ahimsa*). Repeating positive affirmations regularly—such as our foundational affirmation, "I am the mountain. I am stable. I am solid. I am secure. I am balanced" (page 41)—helps replace negative thoughts with positive ones and build our self-confidence and belief in our own abilities.

Through asana, we apply the conscious application of levels of flexibility (see chapter 7) in a mindful way. This approach transforms "can't do" into "can do"—everyone can do any pose at their own level of ability.

What happens when positive thinking is not possible or available to us? We can use the cultivation of opposites to shift into a more *neutral* state, which can move us toward balance and stability in the body-mind. For instance, coming into Sitting Mountain, our foundational pose, asks us to sit actively by engaging the lower-body muscles while relaxing the upper-body muscles, holding the physical body in two opposite states at the same time. Even the two words *active sitting* embody this stance of balancing opposites. Other yoga techniques that take a conscious approach to fostering opposites for balancing the body-mind include Alternate Nostril Breathing (page 64) and a special form of meditation called Yoga Nidra (page 192).

By practicing pratipaksha bhavana, we can train our minds to think more positively and minimize the impact of negative thoughts; we can learn how to balance our body-mind, which can reduce suffering, for the benefit of our happiness and well-being. Our compassion-based chair-yoga approach helps teachers and practitioners gain the skills they need to turn negatives into positives.

Abundance (*Lakshmi*)

During her yoga training, Lakshmi was given the spiritual Sanskrit name Mahalakshmi, with *maha* meaning "great" and *lakshmi* representing the Hindu goddess of abundance, who brings wealth, power, and prosperity. This goddess is known to bestow wisdom, strength, beauty, and a sense of sovereignty to everyone. Our approach to chair yoga honors her legacy by sharing an abundance of knowledge and skills with its teachers and students and encouraging them to pass this richness on to others. By offering access to this fullness of learning, wealth of skills, and depth of inspiration to everyone—regardless of age, ability, or physical or mental condition—this approach ensures that yoga in its entirety is truly inclusive and accessible.

Applying Patanjali's Eight Limbs of Yoga to Chair Yoga

Now that we've covered the key philosophical concepts that are the basis for our chair-yoga practice, let's consider how they might apply to each stage of Patanjali's yogic path. No matter how we interact with yoga—as student or teacher—we can make this path our own, entering wherever suits us and following whichever limbs work for us on our journey.

The first two limbs cover the yamas (the five social restraints) and the niyamas (the five personal observances). All ten yamas and niyamas guide us to right action on and off the chair. They help us to understand the power of right speech—that is, the way we talk to and about ourselves and others (*matrika shakti*)—and the importance of developing our true identity (*sat nam*). They guide teachers to bring their authentic self to the chair, teaching from their love and experience of yoga. And they also encourage students to bring their whole selves to the practice, with kindness and patience.

The third limb covers asana. This is where all the poses come to us in multiple levels of flexibility.

The fourth limb is about pranayama, the gift of proper breathing techniques for the health and well-being of our physical and mental bodies as well as our spiritual life energy.

The fifth limb covers pratyahara, the withdrawal of the external senses, tuning in to our higher self for the guidance of our body without thought. This is where the Sun and Moon Salutations come into play, allowing the body to move easily and effortlessly through the salutation, tapping into our own inner wisdom.

The sixth limb is focused concentration, or dharana. The mind is cleared through pranayama and pratyahara, the flow of our chair-yoga practice is achieved at our own level of flexibility, and sat-chit-ananda—the cycle of life—is acknowledged.

The seventh limb is meditation, or dhyana—which in our approach is part of every chair-yoga class or session. Asanas and pranayama are followed by relaxation or meditation or simply coming into Sitting Mountain for a moment of reflection.

The eighth and last limb is samadhi—enlightenment. Finding joy whenever we take part in or teach chair yoga.

We are humbled every time we sit up on a chair! The seat of the chair is the firm foundation upon which we sit. The front legs of the chair represent the stability of our legs and feet, and the two back chair legs represent the grounding of our sit bones. Each leg of the chair also symbolizes a vital yogic element of support: the yamas, the niyamas, matrika shakti, and sat-chit-ananda. Get fit where you sit—on any chair, anywhere!

4

Levels of Flexibility

You must find the place inside yourself where nothing is impossible.

—DEEPAK CHOPRA

MOST YOGA TEACHERS like to offer their students various ways to make poses easier to execute. Often they begin with what they deem the "fullest expression" of a pose (what the pose is "supposed" to look like) and then give instructions for "modifying the pose" so that it would work for students with different abilities. The problem, of course, is that there is no such thing as the "fullest expression" of a pose. What we see in books, magazines, and social media may look "picture perfect," but the fact is, it's not available to many people. In reality, there's no such thing as a single full expression; one person's pose may look entirely different than another person's. Why? Because every *body* is different; every person has a different level of flexibility (or range of motion).

In our approach to chair yoga, we have a unique way of working with levels of flexibility, which has proven to be quite effective. We like to begin with the very *basic* aspect of a pose—sitting up on a chair, grounding the energy—and then build the pose according to what the body is capable of in that moment. That way, everyone starts at the same place and then goes on to explore, find (and benefit from) their own full expression—without feeling as though they are incapable of doing someone else's idea of the "perfect" pose. This approach makes yoga fully accessible to everyone; it is entirely consistent with "Do no harm"—the yoga concept of ahimsa and the Hippocratic oath taken by doctors in the West; and it offers everyone a chance to strengthen the body-mind connection by encouraging each person to find their own level of practice and gain a sense of ownership of the self. Our approach is truly person-centered, adaptive yoga.

When working with levels of flexibility to adapt poses, keep these key points in mind:

- There will most likely be varying degrees of flexibility in the different planes of the body: the upper and lower body, the front and back body, and the right and left sides of the body.

- Your level of flexibility may vary from day to day. It is therefore important to always start with the most basic posture options so you can find the one that is suitable for you on any given day.

- Chapter 7 outlines our step-by-step approach to adapting poses. Once you understand how to adapt poses safely and appropriately, we encourage you to use your sat nam and creativity to come up with your own options to further inspire and benefit yourself and, if teaching, the audience you serve.

- Practice compassion on the chair: Levels of flexibility allow us to choose what works for us on any given day. It's not about pushing ourselves into what we believe we can do (or should be able to do) if our body is telling us otherwise; it's about recognizing and accepting that each day, each week, each month, each year may be different, giving each of us permission to do yoga our own personal way.

Multiple Levels of Flexibility

How many levels of flexibility are there? While we mainly present three levels of flexibility for the poses in this book, there are often many possibilities. To explain what we mean, let's look at Tree Pose (Vrikshasana). In chapter 9, we present three variations for Tree Pose on a single chair (page 163) and three variations on a wheelchair (pages 164–65), beginning with option A (one example of a basic level of flexibility), followed by option B (an adaptation somewhere in between) and option C (one example of a full expression). The photos in this chapter show *multiple* levels of flexibility, illustrating six different Tree Pose variations, also starting with a basic version, then working up to more extended versions.

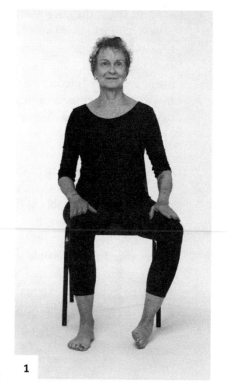

1

(right and next page) Tree Pose variations 1-6

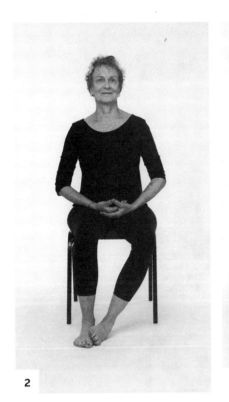

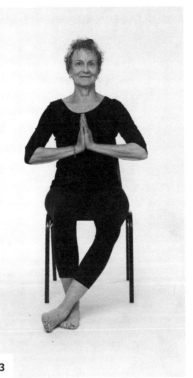

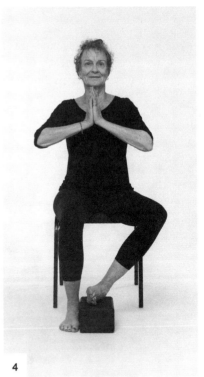

2

3

4

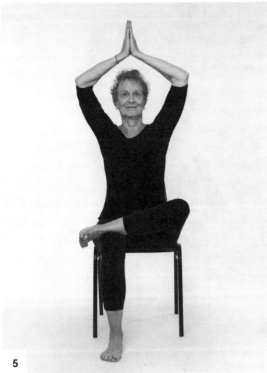

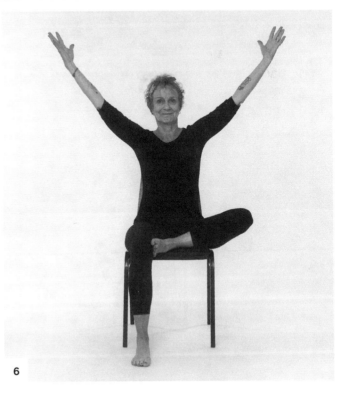

5

6

Mix and Match Levels of Flexibility

What if someone wants to do a particular level with the arms but a different level with the legs? It's perfectly fine—always feel free to mix and match! The photos here offer four Tree Pose variations illustrating ways to choose different levels for the lower and upper body, combining what works based on how a person feels on the day.

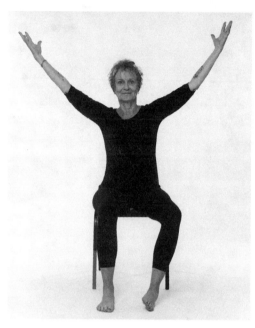

Tree Pose with lower body 1 and upper body 6

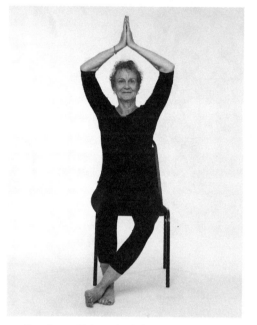

Tree Pose with lower body 3 and upper body 5

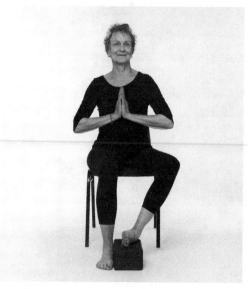

Tree Pose with lower body 4 and upper body 3

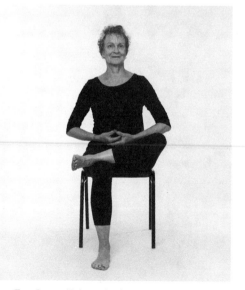

Tree Pose with lower body 5 and upper body 2

Visualization as a Level of Flexibility

The three levels of flexibility we present in this book are all related to range of motion in the physical body. What happens when moving the physical body is not available? Then consider a level of flexibility for the mind: visualization.

Visualization is commonly used in sports training, and scientific evidence shows that just thinking about movement can improve muscle function. Even more than that, visualizing a body part moving can activate the same area of the brain that fires when we are actually moving, which strengthens the body, the brain, and the connection between them. When we *imagine* doing Tree Pose, for instance, we activate muscle fibers that can make muscles stronger and movement more fluid and accurate. To access these benefits, picture yourself doing any physical level of flexibility and visualize engaging the muscles necessary in each step.

Visualization can also help reduce stress, improve concentration, and strengthen the ability to remain in the present moment. Ancient and modern-day yoga practices encourage practitioners to focus using their "inner eye," also called the "Third Eye" (see chapter 6). We suggest how to incorporate visualization into our foundation pose, Sitting Mountain (chapter 5); breathing practices (chapter 8); asana practice (chapter 9); meditation, relaxation, and mindfulness (chapter 10); and other yoga techniques (chapter 12).

Tips for Teaching Levels of Flexibility

When teaching our method of chair yoga, go slow, breathe, and be aware of the levels of flexibility for each asana. Be sure to give your students permission to do each movement or pose at their own level.

Remember to mix and match! Offer students the option of choosing one level for their lower body and a different one for their upper body, or for the different sides of their body, if that's what feels right for them at that moment.

Include visualization as a level of flexibility for the mind, along with levels of flexibility for the body. Provide suggestions to guide students and also encourage them to come up with their own mental images if they wish.

Levels of flexibility ensure that no student has to remain idle during a class—everyone gets to participate! Remind students that no matter the level of flexibility they are practicing, they are receiving all the health and wellness benefits of the practice.

A fun way to apply your sat nam when using our levels of flexibility within a pose might be to choose inventive, nonjudgmental words like *mild*, *medium*, and *spicy* (levels of hotness in salsa); or *bud*, *blossom*, and *flower* (levels of growth for a flower). Feel free to come up with metaphors that speak to you (and your students, if you teach)!

Remind your students (and yourself): "Your body has wisdom—listen to it."

5

Sitting Mountain: The Foundation

I am the mountain. I am stable. I am solid. I am secure. I am balanced.

—LAKSHMI VOELKER

SITTING MOUNTAIN is the foundational pose for our approach to chair yoga. It is the most important pose for learning to sit actively and the one we return to throughout every chair-yoga practice. The Sitting Mountain affirmation above, inspired by Thich Nhat Hạnh from his celebrated book *Peace Is Every Step: The Path of Mindfulness in Everyday Life*, provides a positive statement to match and support our physical movement, reinforcing the body-mind connection.

We always begin a chair-yoga session with Sitting Mountain. Setting our foundation in this way allows us to center and stabilize ourselves, grounding firmly into the earth, actively engaging the lower body. At the same time, it encourages us to lengthen the spine and lift the chest, bringing space between the vertebrae and in the torso and lungs, allowing more freedom for the breath. We come into Sitting Mountain—the pose itself as well as each cue—with mindful movement, a reminder for us to pay attention to our posture and realign as needed. Sitting Mountain is a signal that it's time to come into our yoga space.

Below are step-by-step instructions for teaching and practicing Sitting Mountain safely and effectively, laying the groundwork for learning how to adapt any yoga pose. Because this pose is so important, we explain the cues in great detail. When doing it for the first time, a good way to learn Sitting Mountain is to follow each of these steps with care and attention. Take a few moments to mindfully practice each cue and ask yourself, "How does Sitting Mountain feel in my body?" We encourage you to play with it! Once you find Sitting Mountain in your own body, there is no need to go through all these steps every time you sit on a chair. Once you know Sitting Mountain, simply remind yourself (or your students) of a few cues that are most important to you. Each person will find their own way of sitting actively in Sitting Mountain that works for them.

First, choose a chair that is safe, secure, and adjusted to suit your body. Use props as needed so you can sit toward the front edge of the chair in good postural alignment. For example, you may need blocks under your feet so your thighs are parallel to the ground, a cushion behind your back to sit forward with a lengthened spine, or a blanket under your buttocks to raise your torso if your knees are higher than your hips. For considerations when choosing a chair and for tips on how to use props to adapt any chair to suit any *body*, see chapter 12.

These instructions can be used as a script for your own practice or for teaching students when they are first learning how to do Sitting Mountain. You will find levels of flexibility and further tips for Sitting Mountain in chapter 9 (see Mountain Pose on page 142). See chapter 6 for further details of key alignment principles for Sitting Mountain and other poses.

SITTING MOUNTAIN
Step-by-Step Instructions

Sit on a stable and secure chair with your feet flat on the ground. Beginning with the lower-body foundation—the base of the mountain—move forward so that your buttocks are safely as close to the front edge of the chair seat as possible; that way you'll have some space behind you, and your upper body (torso) will be at a right angle with your thighs.

Place your right hand under your right buttock, feeling for the bone in the center (the sit bone). Stay there for one breath and then slide your hand out toward the side. Repeat on the left. This grounding technique anchors and stabilizes you on the chair.

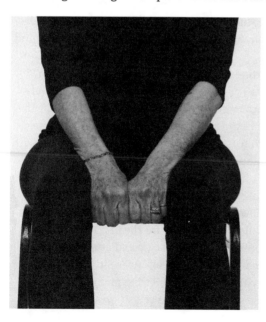

Make two fists, palms down and knuckles facing up, and place them side by side between your knees. Move your fists up between your thighs, drawing them into the soft tissue between your thighs. This will bring your hip bones (pelvis) into proper hip alignment. Adjust your feet as needed so that your hips, knees, and ankles are aligned at right angles.

Place your feet parallel to each other, with the second toe of each foot facing forward in the same direction as your knees. Lift your toes, pushing down firmly to engage the three press points in the soles of your feet: two in the balls of your feet—one in line with your big toe and

Fists placed between thighs for hip alignment

one in line with your little toe—and one in the center of your heel; imagine these points are like the roots of a tree. This automatically creates a proper pelvic tilt. Release your toes down, keeping your feet and leg muscles engaged; imagine you are going to stand up while remaining seated on your chair.

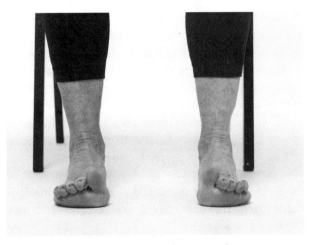

Feet parallel, toes lifted, three press points engaged

Now for the upper-body alignment. Bring the thumb and index finger of one hand together, touching them below your belly button (navel), and rest your other hand on your leg. Imagine you are holding the tab of a zipper and slowly zipping a jacket up the front of your body. As you do so, you'll draw your attention to lengthening the front of your body, making space between your pelvis and ribs and between your hips and armpits. Moving up the front of your body, you'll lift your chest (sternum), which will broaden the space between your shoulder blades (scapulae) in the midback (thoracic vertebrae) and your collarbones (clavicles) in the front on top of your shoulders, relaxing the muscles of your rib cage (intercostals) and opening your heart.

Moving up toward your throat, make a fist and place it in the hollow of your neck. Rest your chin on your little finger. This will bring your head into proper alignment, lengthening your neck and upper back (cervical vertebrae). Release your fist.

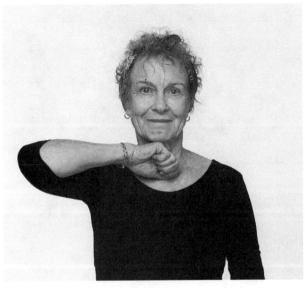
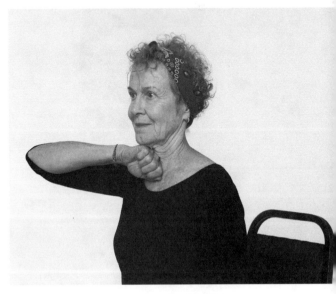

Fist placed under chin for head alignment

Place your tongue gently against the roof of your mouth (soft palate), with the tip behind the back of your front teeth, and swallow once. Lift the crown of your head (the place between the back of your head and your forehead at the top of your skull), keeping your chin parallel to the ground, and sit up tall. Rest your hands on your thighs.

Now, visualize the zipper traveling down your back body to your lower (lumbar) spine, anchoring your sacrum and tailbone (coccyx), allowing the back of your body to lengthen. Relax your arms down by your sides, palms facing forward and thumbs turned back as far as is comfortable for your rotator cuff, opening your shoulders.

Roll your shoulders up, back, and down, without collapsing into your chest or rounding your shoulders. Bring your hands to your thighs or knees, thumb and index finger touching in the hand gesture called Jnana Mudra (palms facing up) or Chin Mudra (palms facing down). Softly extend the other three fingers on each hand, representing sat-chit-ananda.

Make sure your upper body and lower body are in right-angle alignment to one another, as if you are sitting up with your back against a wall. You take on the same shape as the chair on which you are sitting. Close your eyes or choose a place to focus your eyes (*drishti*) with a soft gaze.

Repeat the Sitting Mountain affirmation: "I am the mountain. I am stable. I am solid. I am secure. I am balanced." Inhale and exhale through your nose, becoming aware of your breath. Continue to breathe naturally or consciously alter your breath using a technique of your choice (see chapter 8).

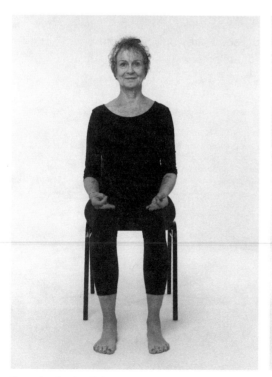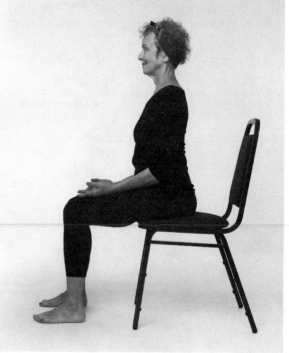

Example of active Sitting Mountain, front view (left) and side view (right). See further views and levels of flexibility in Chapter 9 (page 143).

Now you are in Sitting Mountain. Imagine magnets pulling in opposite directions: the crown of your head being pulled up to the heavens, and your sit bones and the soles of your feet being pulled down onto the earth. Your lower-body muscles are engaged, and your upper-body muscles are relaxed. You are now sitting up (not down) on the chair. This is active sitting.

Sitting *down* loads the spine and the nervous system, while sitting *up* lifts and opens the spine as well as the lungs and diaphragm so that newly oxygenated blood can flow freely to the brain and the body. Sitting up in Sitting Mountain allows the spine to lengthen; we prefer to cue the spine to lengthen rather than straighten to encourage the spine's natural curves to come into play. It also allows the breath to flow naturally and do its job of calming or energizing, as we wish, bringing balance to mood as well as posture.

When any of the Sitting Mountain cues are not possible or available, visualize instead. By visualizing or imagining the movements, the corresponding areas of your brain responsible for these actions are also activated, thereby allowing you to gain the benefits of active sitting.

Sitting Mountain embodies three holistic principles developed by Vanda Scaravelli, author of *Awakening the Spine* and student of the influential yoga teachers B. K. S. Iyengar and T. K. V. Desikachar. It uses gravity and the activation of the muscles to make the pose stable. By lifting the chest, anchoring the sit bones, and supporting postural balance, Sitting Mountain lengthens the spine from this stable base. And it enables the breath to flow freely, which releases the spine so that it can lengthen and extend. In Sitting Mountain, you can feel the flow of energy as it moves through the body—grounding down, lengthening, rising up—and you are encouraged to find that perfect balance in your body-mind between effort and ease.

QUICK GUIDE TO SITTING MOUNTAIN CUES AND POSTURAL ALIGNMENT

1. Come forward toward front edge of chair seat.

2. Anchor sit bones.

3. Position legs hip-width apart (hip alignment).

4. Check for right angles at hips, knees, and ankles.

5. Ensure feet are parallel facing in same direction as knees (foot alignment).

6. Engage three press points in feet.

7. Lengthen the front of the body.

8. Lift and expand chest.

9. Position chin parallel to the ground.

10. Gently place tongue on roof of mouth.

11. Lift crown of head (head alignment).

12. Lengthen the back of the body.

13. Rotate shoulders up, back, and down.

14. Place palms facing up or down.

15. Focus.

16. Repeat Sitting Mountain affirmation.

17. Find your own Sitting Mountain. Breathe.

Tips for Teaching Sitting Mountain

In addition to starting and ending your practice with Sitting Mountain, you can use this posture as a transition between poses, movements, and other yoga techniques. Come back to Sitting Mountain throughout your yoga practice to pause, rest, and reset your body, mind, and breath.

Feel free to modify the Sitting Mountain cues above, choosing what works best for you and your students. For instance, a variation for the lower body when the thighs fully touch and the knees face outward in a V shape is to bring the heels in line with each other and the knees over the ankles, allowing the feet to point in the same direction as the knees before lifting the toes and engaging the three press points. An alternative to placing the fist in the hollow of the neck for head alignment is to press two fingers onto the chin to bring it down, up, or back into a position parallel to the ground, or simply visualize this.

Repeat the Sitting Mountain affirmation. When teaching it, have practitioners repeat the statement in full after you say it, in parts in the manner of a call-and-response, or silently to themselves. Another descriptive affirmation that our students and teachers love is: "Sit taller, as tall as the trees on top of the mountain." Feel free to modify these affirmations or come up with your own.

Remember to come into Sitting Mountain any time during the day to unload stress from the spine (for good physical health) and the nervous system (for good mental health).

6

Principles of Alignment

Lengthen, strengthen, extend, expand.

—LAKSHMI VOELKER

FOCUSING ON THE principles of alignment allows us to practice in a manner that creates ease and spaciousness in the whole body. Postural alignment affords us the opportunity to lengthen, strengthen, extend, and expand the body, helping to maintain and/or improve health and wellness. Paying attention to proper alignment also ensures security and safety, prime considerations for every yoga practice (see chapter 12). Using our levels of flexibility makes these benefits of alignment more accessible to and safer for more people.

Although good posture and postural alignment begin physically with the feet, we will start at the top of the body, working our way down, to explain the key alignment principles and safety components.

Focus of the Eyes (*Drishti*) and Neck Safety

The focused gaze of the eyes—our drishti—is important for helping find balance and steadiness, improve alignment, maintain concentration and focus, and enhance alertness and awareness. We offer many options to choose from.

Drishti can be directed to the high seam—the space where the wall and the ceiling meet—or to the low seam—where the wall meets the floor—or anywhere in between. It can also be directed anywhere from the low seam along the floor to the feet or the legs. This all depends on the asana we are practicing and our level of flexibility in the moment. The eyes may be closed or half-open with a soft downward gaze.

In Sitting Mountain, we can look straight ahead (keeping the chin parallel to the ground) or lower the eyes just a bit.

In poses where we wish to look up, we gaze upward toward the high seam (depending on the height of the ceiling) but no higher, to protect the neck from stretching back too far and to avoid pinching the vertebral arteries and nerves in the neck and at the base of the skull. Such backward movement risks restricting blood flow (and oxygen) to the brain, which could result in numbness, dizziness, weakness, or arm challenges. We never advocate dropping or rolling the head all the way back—or looking up at the ceiling—with our upward drishti. Instead, we encourage lengthening the back of the neck, lifting the chin slightly, opening the throat, and imagining that the head is being cradled or supported.

Other options for drishti include looking down at the ground; focusing on the floor a few feet in front of us; or bringing the gaze to the toes or legs. Drishti allows us to focus inward as well—on the space between the eyebrows, called the "Third Eye." It's not necessary to close the eyes—some people find that to be uncomfortable; keeping them open with a downward gaze and a soft focus is absolutely fine.

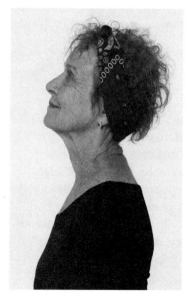
High-seam drishti

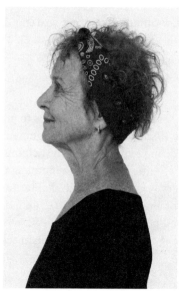
Forward drishti

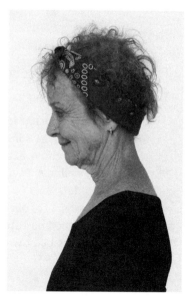
Low-seam drishti

Arm Raising and Lowering, and Shoulder Safety

The shoulder is a complex joint that includes the rotator cuff and acromion bone. Raising and lowering your arms properly is important for keeping both shoulders safe. Proper movement of the arms and hands helps free the rotator cuff and put the acromion process—the bony bit that sticks out from the top of your shoulder—in alignment with the rotator. It also helps prevent shoulder impingement syndrome, in which the tendons of the rotator and subacromial bursa are pinched in the narrow space beneath the acromion bone, becoming inflamed and swollen.

HOW TO SAFELY RAISE AND LOWER YOUR ARMS FROM THE SIDES OF YOUR BODY

Place your arms down by your sides with your palms facing inward. Raise your arms halfway up and, when they reach shoulder height, rotate your hands at your wrists to turn your palms upward. Then, if available, continue to raise your arms up as high as is comfortable, palms facing inward. When bringing your arms down, keep your palms facing inward. When your arms reach shoulder height, rotate your hands so your palms face downward. Then bring your arms down by your sides. This method is particularly important to use when your arms are fully straightened out to shoulder height with no bend in your elbows.

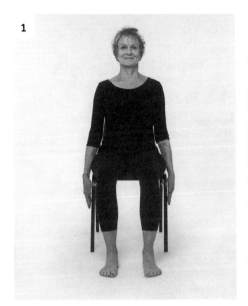

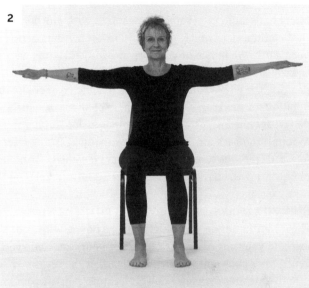

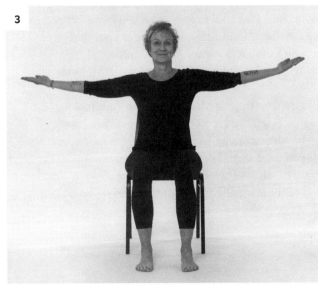

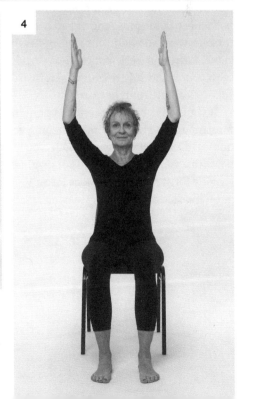

1. Start with arms by side, palms inward
2. Raise arms to shoulder height, palms down
3. Rotate palms up
4. Raise arms overhead, palms inward. Reverse movement to lower arms.

Important: When raising your arms up from the sides of your body—in a pose such as Tree Pose—or to the front—in Chair Pose, for example—keep your shoulders relaxed and only raise your arms as high as is comfortable without tensing and hiking them up toward your ears. If your blood pressure is not well controlled, be sure to keep your head level, your neck in line with your spine, and your gaze forward (not upward) when raising your arms to avoid lightheadedness or dizziness.

Forward Folding from the Hips and Spinal Safety

Many of us sit (and in some cases, stand) with our necks too far forward, increasing the hump in the midback (thoracic spine) and inverting the pelvic region, which can negatively affect our health. We hunch or curl forward while driving, working on our computers, or relaxing on the couch; hardly anyone sits up straight when using their cell phones. With this forward-head posture, the whole body is off-balance, which can create neck, back, and hip challenges. Bending forward can exacerbate these challenges, which is particularly problematic for anyone with bone loss, osteoporosis, spinal fusion, or any spinal disc conditions. We don't want to round the back any more than it already is. Instead, we want to retrain the body to hinge forward from the hips, so that the torso *lengthens*, bringing space between the vertebrae while maintaining the natural curves in the spine and keeping the back safe.

HOW TO SAFELY HINGE FORWARD FROM THE HIPS
Place your hands on your thighs, palms down, with your thumbs resting on the inside of your legs and your fingers on the outside of your legs. Slide your hands up to the crease between your upper body and your legs. Squeeze at the crease, or simply press your thumbs or fingers into the hip crease to feel your hips. Sit up tall, lift your chest, dip your chin slightly, and, leading with your ribs and chest, hinge forward from your hips, lengthening the front of your body. Keep your spine lengthened, strengthened, extended, and expanded as you move your torso forward and find your level of flexibility—without rounding in any part of your middle spine. Keep your neck and cervical vertebrae, which are an extension of your spine, in line with your spine. Practice hinging forward and then backward from your hips with this long spine, "leading from the heart."

If your lower back or sacrum is tight, make circles with your torso or tilt your hips (pelvis) forward and back a few times, keeping your spine lengthened, before you hinge. If you have uncontrolled blood pressure, move slowly and be sure not to let your head drop below your heart to avoid lightheadedness or dizziness. If you need to make space for the belly when hinging forward, bring the legs into a V-shaped or L-shaped position when facing forward or on the side of your chair (see an explanation of these leg alignment alternatives below on page 52).

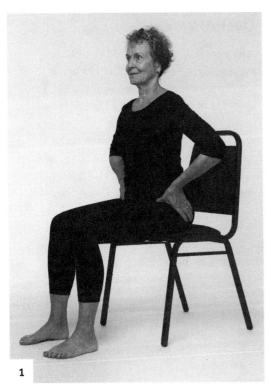

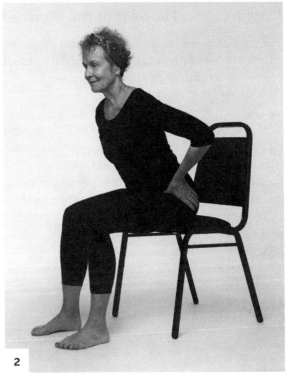

1. Sit up tall with spine lengthened

2. Hinge forward from hips with spine lengthened

3. Hinge back from hips with spine lengthened

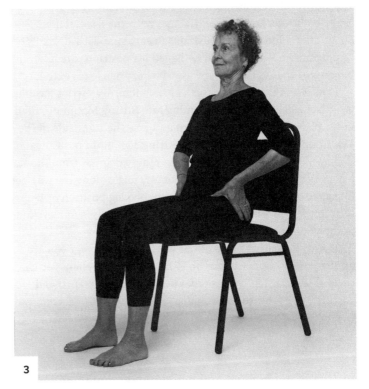

The Seat of the Chair and Overall Safety

The ideal chair will support good postural alignment. While our chair-yoga method can be adapted to any chair, a chair seat that is flat or tilted down slightly at the front will help to promote a neutral hip position. (See chapter 12 for more on chair safety.) The connection of our sit bones to the seat of the chair also serves as another point of grounding, in addition to the feet connecting us to the earth.

When moving into and out of poses, especially those we do when sitting to face toward the right or left side of the chair, we can use the seat for safety and balance by holding the front, side, or back edges. Holding the seat edge rather than the back of the chair prevents us from hiking up the shoulders, which can put undue pressure on the neck and shoulders. Using the seat edge to adjust our position helps remind us to keep the shoulders down and relaxed.

To ensure proper postural alignment when a chair seat is too high or too low, we can add props under the feet or the buttocks (to raise or lower the legs into right angles). Props can be used in this way from the start of a session, or they can be added at the end for practitioners whose feet dangle when sitting back on the seat during meditation or relaxation. With the use of props, any chair can be adapted to suit *any* body!

Leg Alignment Alternatives: V-Shaped Leg, L-Shaped Leg, and Extended Leg

For some postures, such as Triangle Pose and many of the Warrior poses, the position of the lower body—as practiced on the mat with the leg extended—is not available to everyone. So we offer additional leg positions to accommodate all levels of flexibility and to avoid hip impingement. V-shaped and L-shaped leg positions are alternative ways to safely receive the benefits of these poses (or any asana where one leg is extended back).

How does this work in practice? Let's look at Warrior I as illustrated in the photos here (see also page 175). Begin by coming into Sitting Mountain, then set up the position of your lower body for a stable base. Turn and face the right side of the chair and reestablish Sitting Mountain. Keep your right leg in Sitting Mountain position and slide open your left leg into a V-shaped leg position, moving up to ninety degrees from the stable right leg into an L-shaped leg position. Your left leg can stop at any angle along the way between Sitting Mountain and L-shaped leg position. Remain in V-shaped leg position or L-shaped leg position or lengthen your left leg back into an extended leg position (see foot alignment below) before going on to set up your upper body.

These alternative leg positions work well wherever you are seated on the chair and setting up the pose—at the front or on either side of the chair. See chapter 9 for step-by-step instructions of Warrior I as well as other poses where V-shaped and L-shaped legs help make the postures accessible to everyone.

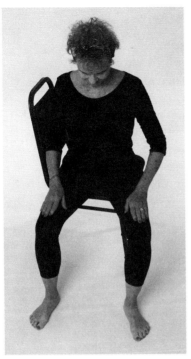

V-shaped leg as viewed from above

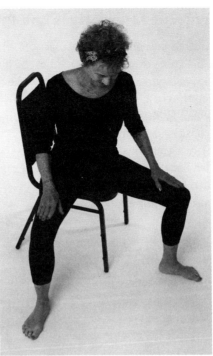

L-shaped leg as viewed from above

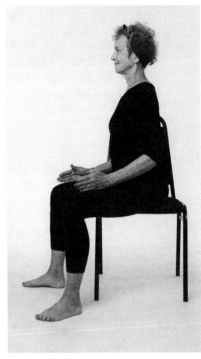

V-shaped leg in Warrior I

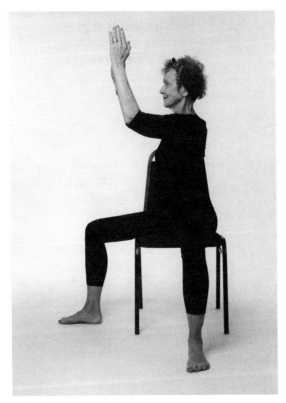

L-shaped leg in Warrior I

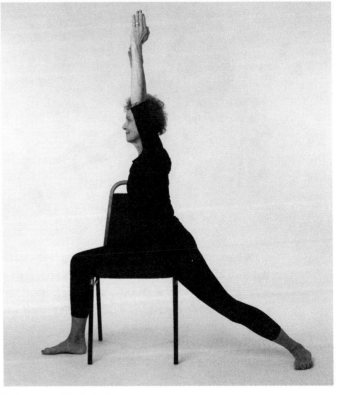

Extended leg in Warrior I

Foot Alignment Alternatives and Press Points

In Sitting Mountain, we bring our feet into a parallel position, with right angles at the ankles so that the heels are under the knees to assist alignment of the hips, which in turn allows support for spinal and upper-body alignment. What happens to the feet in postures such as High Lunge Pose and Warrior II on the chair?

We first offer to keep the feet in Sitting Mountain. Or you can bring your legs and feet into a V-shaped or L-shaped leg position as outlined above. In all these positions, your feet are pointing in the same direction as your knees.

When your leg is extended back in poses such as High Lunge Pose (see here and on page 175), the foot of your extended leg comes onto the front two press points in the ball of your foot and the heel presses back while remaining lifted.

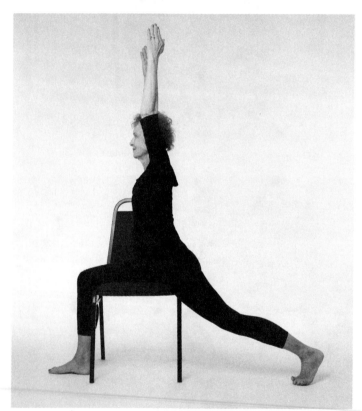

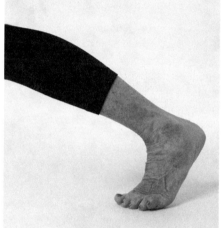

(above) Extended leg on ball of foot

(left) Extended leg in High Lunge Pose

When your leg is extended back in poses such as Warrior II (see here and on page 179), the foot of your extended leg moves and realigns when your body is turning. In practice, one way to do this is to extend the back leg from an L-shaped leg position, allowing the heel of your back foot to swivel away and lie flat. Or if your leg is extended onto the ball of the back foot, let your heel turn inward and drop down to lie flat (please do not remain on the ball of the foot). Your toes will then point forward and the energy will be transferred to the outside (little-toe side) of your foot.

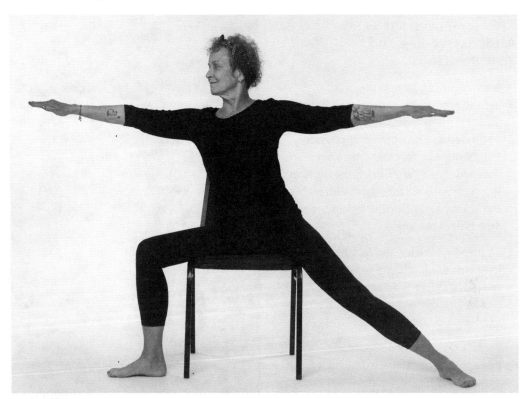

(above) Extended leg in Warrior II

(left) Extended leg with turned foot and sole flat

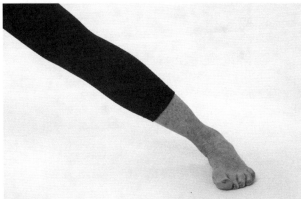

Inspired by Kripalu's press-point system,[9] we encourage a dynamic use of press points in the feet to assist in supporting postural alignment for stability, building strength in the lower body, and fostering focus in both body and mind. Once the feet are aligned, we push the press points in the feet firmly down onto the ground—this engages the arches of the feet as well as the muscles of the lower body. In poses where the sole of the foot is fully in contact with the ground, there are three press points: one in the heel and two in the ball of the foot (one in line with the big toe and the other in line with the little toe). For those poses where the heel is lifted, such as High Lunge Pose, only the two press points in the ball of the foot are engaged.

Tips for Poses with Alternative Leg and Feet Positions

- Start in Sitting Mountain—a parallel leg and foot position is the most basic aspect for most poses and should always be offered as a first option. If physically the thighs fully touch and the knees face outward in a V shape, bring the heels in line with each other, align the knees over the ankles, and point the feet in the same direction as the knees.

- Be sure that the leg and foot that remain in Sitting Mountain are secure and grounded before moving into more challenging options with the other leg and foot.

- Explore the various V-shaped and L-shaped leg positions, extended leg options, and foot alternatives to find what's most suitable and safe on a given day.

- For further examples of poses with alternative leg and feet positions, see chapter 9.

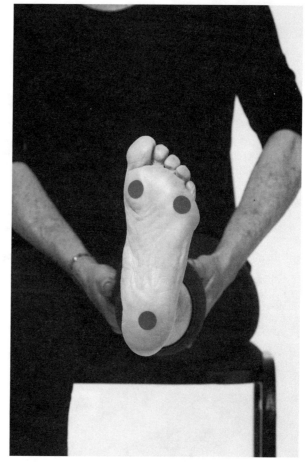

Three press points in each foot

7

Adapting Poses to the Chair

Adapt the asana to your body where it is today, right now, with no judgment
or expectation. Let the body be in its present moment.

—LAKSHMI VOELKER

BELOW ARE STEP-BY-STEP instructions for how to adapt any pose effectively and safely,
using our levels of flexibility and learning how to "feel" into each pose. Before you start, it
is important to approach the process of adapting a pose to the chair with an open mind, a
"beginner's mind"—as if you are coming to yoga for the very first time. This chapter will
get you started. You'll find more resources in part three (beginning on page 61) and a list of
teachers and training courses for the Lakshmi Voelker Method available via our website.

How to Cultivate a Beginner's Mind

For those who are new to yoga, you already have beginner's mind! For those who have been
practicing or teaching yoga for a long time, the body and mind will have stored particular
patterns, images, and memories of what yoga is, what it looks like, how it's done. That might
mean an expression of a pose that, for many people, is just not possible or available. By accessing your beginner's mind, you can practice or present a pose in new and flexible ways that are
available to any and every *body*.

How do we go about cultivating a beginner's mind? Think of something you did for the first
time. For instance, take yourself back to the first time you did yoga. Or the first time you rode
a bike, drove a car, started a new job, or held your newborn child or grandchild in your arms.
What was it like? How did it feel? Were you nervous or excited? Was it joyful or scary? When

you bring this first-ever experience to mind, you remember what it feels like to approach something brand-new, free from ingrained habits or preconceived notions. When you do that, you're making room for new learning—taking off one hat and putting on another. Now, take a deep breath, exhale completely, and get ready to learn how to adapt a pose the Lakshmi Voelker Method way.

ADAPTING A POSE TO THE CHAIR

Step-by-Step Instructions

1. Choose an asana on the mat that you want to adapt. (Can't think of one? Check out the forty poses in chapter 9.)

2. Come into the pose on the mat. If you are unable to access the mat, come into the pose on a chair—or simply visualize doing it. Remember that the chair version won't necessarily look the same as the traditional mat pose because you're adapting it for the chair, not the mat. But it should *feel* the same in your body. Notice how the pose feels in your body.

3. Ask yourself, "What is my intention? What am I trying to achieve?"

4. Look closely at the mat pose and imagine how it might be adapted to a chair. Is it better to face the front of the chair or the side edge? Would it be beneficial to experiment with any tools or props, such as blocks, straps, cushions, or blankets? Be creative! Bring your sat nam—your true authentic self—into the process.

5. Once you have absorbed the feel of the pose on the mat and decided on your intention, sit on the chair and align your body correctly in Sitting Mountain.

6. Now come into *your* full expression of the pose to start the process of adapting. Begin with the lower body, taking the position back a level, then back another level, repeating this until you get to the simplest variation. Then do the same with your upper body. Always be aware of multiple levels as you align your body to match the mat pose *in effect, not look.*

Let's use Tree Pose (Vrikshasana) as an example. Begin in Mountain Pose (Tadasana). Close your eyes and imagine yourself as a strong tree: one leg stable, aligned, and grounded like a tree trunk, the other leg positioned according to your level of flexibility on the stable leg and both arms lifted in the air. Now let's adapt the pose on the chair from the ground up.

Design your lower body first. Begin in Sitting Mountain. Choose one leg to be the stable tree trunk. The other leg can move so your foot is placed on its outside edge or touching your stable leg's foot; or it crosses your stable leg at the ankle; or it is positioned above the knee on the thigh of your stable leg.

Now design your upper body. Place both hands in your lap, cradling one hand into the palm of the other; or bring your palms together at your heart center; or raise both arms overhead far apart or with palms together as available. Voila! We have Tree Pose on the chair with levels of flexibility.

Remember, while Tree Pose on the chair may not look the same as Tree Pose on the mat, the feeling and the benefits are the same. By adapting the pose and employing levels of flexibility, you offer your students the opportunity to find options and make choices that meet their own particular wants, needs, and desires.

Tips for Adapting Asanas

When adapting poses, always start in Sitting Mountain. Set up your lower-body level of flexibility first to establish a safe and solid foundation. Then, while holding your lower-body level of flexibility, set up your upper-body level of flexibility, again backing up the movement if you reach a level that is too challenging.

Keep in mind that each body is different on the left and right sides, in the upper and lower parts, and in the front and back. This is why levels of flexibility are so important. As you move through the levels, if you reach one that presents a challenge, go back to a previous level. Give yourself permission to mix and match, honoring the differing levels of flexibility of your upper and lower body, front and back body, and sides of your body—on that particular day. Remember that each day may be different!

Be clear about your intention (purpose, aim, or goal) for your practice and about the benefits you wish to achieve. Once you come into the variation that works for you, hold the pose for three breaths to activate the asana.

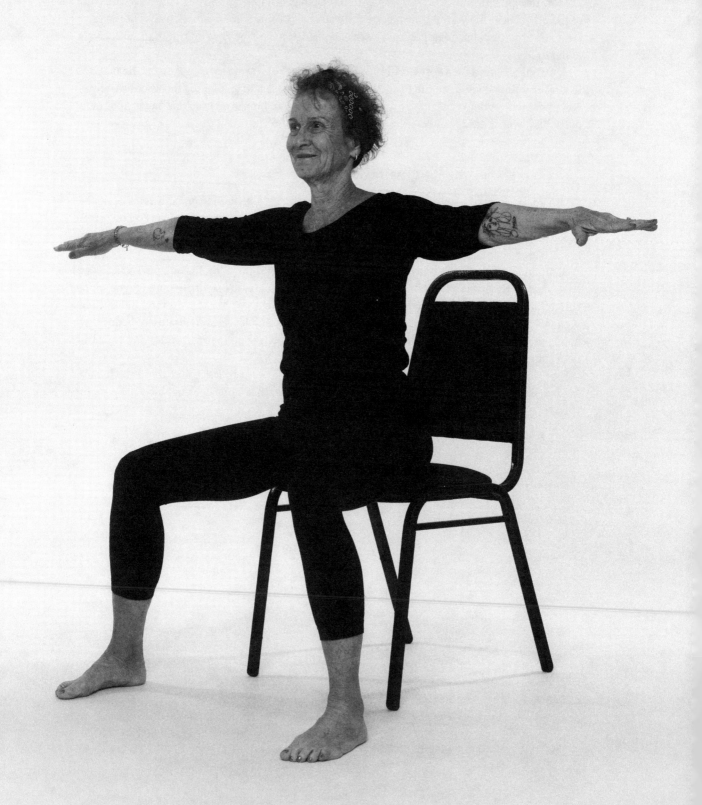

PART THREE

The Fundamentals

8

Six Breathing Techniques

By concentrating on our breathing, "In" and "Out," we bring body and
mind back together, and become whole again.

—THICH NHAT HANH, *Peace Is Every Step*

Yoga is an effortless dance with breath and gravity.

—VANDA SCARAVELLI

IN CHAPTER 1, we covered the importance of active sitting: by purposely sitting up on
our chair, we can align our body in a way that not only lengthens, strengthens, extends, and
expands the spine but also creates space for the breath. Yoga, with its long tradition of pranayama, offers many techniques for exploring the breath, and our approach makes them easily
accessible for everyone.

As with mat yoga, focusing on the breath can be done as a stand-alone (sitting, of course!)
technique; it can be coordinated with movement; and it can be combined with meditation
and relaxation (see page 188 for a meditation that focuses specifically on exploring the breath).
Most pranayamas encourage breathing through the nose rather than the mouth whenever possible, with positive benefits to both physical and mental health, including better functioning
of the respiratory and immune systems, better hydration, decreased nasal congestion, and the
potential to lower anxiety and improve sleep.

We have chosen six breathing techniques that we use regularly on the chair, providing
step-by-step instructions using our levels of flexibility. These include five traditional yoga pranayamas—Alternate Nostril Breathing (Anuloma Viloma/Nadi Shodhana); the cooling breath
practices (Sitali/Sitkari); Humming Bee Breath (Bhramari); Three-Part Breath (Dirgha); and a
warming breath practice, Victorious Breath (Ujjayi)—plus Coherent Breathing.

Each of these breathing techniques allows us to practice consciously controlling our breath
and becoming more aware of it, which fosters better concentration as well as present-moment

attention. These techniques also provide a means of slowing down the breath as well as deepening it, which brings many wellness benefits. Slow and deep breathing helps to stimulate the movement of the diaphragm, massaging the internal organs, toning the abdominal muscles, and activating the parasympathetic nervous system—our rest-and-digest system—which can reduce stress. To bring a sense of calm to your body-mind, simply make your exhalation longer than your inhalation. To energize your body-mind, increase the length of your inhale. To maintain balance in your body-mind, keep the inhalation and the exhalation the same length.

Tips for Practicing Pranayama

When working with your breath, ask yourself, "What is my intention? What am I trying to achieve?" For instance, is the goal to energize? Or is it to relax and calm down? The breathing techniques you choose depend on the benefits you desire and whether you are using pranayama in meditation or in an asana-based session to coordinate breath with movement.

Remember that breathing is the only autonomic (involuntary) function in the body that is under our conscious control, and it is a key tool in helping us develop and access present-moment awareness and mindfulness. When you are focused on your breath, you are fully present in the here and now.

All breathing styles can be adapted to the chair using our levels of flexibility—even pranayama has levels of flexibility. Use your sat nam to explore!

If you have any breathing issues or conditions, the natural breath or the most basic variation of a breathing technique may be the most suitable option. As needed, please check with your doctor or health-care professional for guidance and refer to the precautions under each pranayama in this chapter and in chapter 12.

Alternate Nostril Breathing
(Anuloma Viloma/Nadi Shodhana Pranayama)

Alternate Nostril Breathing is said to balance the breath between the left and right nostrils, slow the breath down, promote openness in the lungs, and bring equilibrium to the nervous system. It involves inhaling and exhaling into each nostril separately in a particular pattern.

Its two Sanskrit names describe different aspects of this ancient practice. *Anuloma viloma* highlights qualities of balancing opposites (*pratipaksha bhavana*) as the breath moves from one nostril to the other—*anuloma* can be translated as "with the grain" and *viloma* as "against the grain"—illustrating the alternating movement between the left and right nostrils and their qualities of calming versus energizing, cooling versus warming, feminine versus masculine. *Nadi shodhana* can be translated as "channel cleaning," which refers to the regular cleansing that occurs during the nasal cycle, a natural shifting between the left and right nostrils; another translation is "cleansing the energy pathways," which describes the cleansing of prana (life-giving force) to restore well-being in the body-mind as the breath alternates from one nostril to the other.

ALTERNATE NOSTRIL BREATHING
How It Works

Breathing through the left nostril generates a sense of calm by activating a relaxation response from the parasympathetic nervous system (rest-and-digest system); left-nostril breathing cools the body and is associated with the right hemisphere of the brain, the calming side of the brain. Breathing through the right nostril stimulates the sympathetic nervous system (fight-or-flight mode); right-nostril breathing energizes the body and is associated with the left hemisphere of the brain.

Traditionally, Alternate Nostril Breathing starts and ends with the left nostril: you begin by breathing into your left nostril and finish the practice by exhaling from your left nostril. If you'd like, you can do it using the classic hand position or by using one or two hands, or by visualizing the movement of your breath—any of these choices can help you control the inhalation and exhalation. The instructions below outline several options, including bringing your hands into Vishnu Mudra, a classic yogic hand sign known as a "gesture of universal balance" (see option C).

The breathing pattern for one round of Alternate Nostril Breathing is as follows: (1) Close your right nostril. (2) Inhale through your left nostril. (3) Close your left nostril. (4) Hold your breath (optional). (5) Open and exhale through your right nostril. (6) Inhale through your right nostril. (7) Close your right nostril. (8) Hold your breath (optional). (9) Open and exhale through your left nostril.

The inhale and exhale are usually kept to the same length; many practitioners also hold their breath briefly at the top of each inhale. This breath retention is believed to strengthen the immune system and increase oxygenation. If you're new to breath practices, are pregnant, or have respiratory conditions, introducing breath retention is best done under the guidance of a teacher or a professional; when in doubt, avoid holding your breath altogether. Instead, simply pause briefly, if that feels appropriate, at the end of the exhale and wait for the inhale to come on its own.

For beginners and those who experience breathlessness, start with a 2:1:2 or 2:2:2 ratio (inhale, pause, exhale), doing just a few rounds, and build from there if available and desired, increasing the ratio and the number of rounds if and when the technique becomes more comfortable. For greater calm, make the exhalation longer than the inhalation. For those with congestion, challenges with the hands, or when touching the face is not available, use visualizations (option A below) to access the benefits of this breathing practice.

"We can find the breath in the space between thoughts, between heartbeats, between muscle and bone."

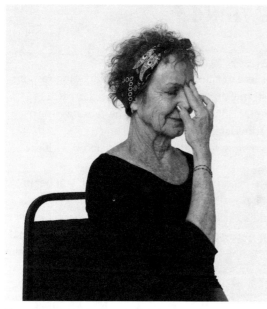

View of Vishnu Mudra from the right in Alternate Nostril Breathing (option C)

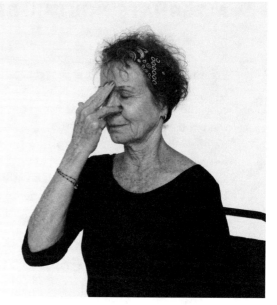

View of Vishnu Mudra from the left in Alternate Nostril Breathing (option C)

Alternate Nostril Breathing: Variations

Come into Sitting Mountain, allowing your eyes to close or softening your gaze. Start with your natural breath, inhaling and exhaling gently through your nose for several breaths. Allow your breath to slow and deepen into your belly. Now choose one of the variations below that works for you in the present moment—or create one of your own.

A. Using visualization: Place your hands onto your lap and visualize your breath coming into your left nostril to begin, then follow the breathing pattern outlined above. To help maintain focus, imagine your breath traveling up the side of a mountain on the inhale and down the other side of the mountain on the exhale, or come up with your own visualization.

B. Using two hands: Use the index fingers of each hand to open and close your nostrils, following the breathing pattern outlined above.

C. Using one hand (Vishnu Mudra): Use only your right hand to open and close your nostrils. Your index and middle fingers can touch the space between your eyebrows—the "Third Eye"—or curl into the palm of your hand in Vishnu Mudra. Use your right thumb to close your right nostril and your right ring and little fingers to close your left nostril. Follow the breathing pattern outlined above. (See the photos above for reference.)

Duration: Continue for as many rounds as you wish, finishing by exhaling from your left nostril to keep your body-mind cool and balanced. At the end of the practice, rest your hands on your thighs and return to your natural breath.

Cooling Breath (Sitali/Sitkari)

The cooling breath practices are said to reduce heat and induce calm by cooling the body in hot weather and from hot flashes (e.g., in menopause or chemotherapy treatment) as well as cooling feelings of frustration, anger, or rage; strengthen the tongue; and support good postural alignment of the head and neck. They involve drawing the breath in over the tongue with the mouth open (on the inhale only). *Sitali* means "cooling" or "soothing," while *Sitkari* means "sipping" or "hissing." Each Sanskrit name indicates a different option, a clear indication that the ancient yogis believed in creating "levels of flexibility" to make this pranayama accessible to all!

COOLING BREATH

How It Works

In the practice of Sitali, the tongue is curled, with the sides of the tongue rolled upward into a tube shape (see option A). A curled tongue is not genetically possible for everyone, so Sitkari offers a variation where the tongue is extended over the bottom lip (see option B). If you have sensitive teeth or if the traditional cooling breath practices cause discomfort, there's a third option in which the tip of the tongue is placed behind the upper teeth (see option C).

In all variations, the inhalation is moistened as it passes through the curl or over the surface of the tongue. The action of the tongue can also be described as akin to a bird feeding with its beak, "drinking" water-saturated air on the inhale, and an uncurling leaf as the tongue returns inside on the exhale. Between the inhale and exhale, you can hold or pause your breath briefly (optional) in order to retract the tongue and close the mouth, enhancing the mindfulness of the practice.

Please note that the cooling breath is one of the few yoga breathing techniques when mouth breathing is used—but only on the inhale, not on the exhale. Inhaling through the mouth can sometimes cause dryness, which may lead to coughing or discomfort. If this is the case, take a few sips of water before or during the practice as needed, and keep the number of rounds to just a few breaths.

Cooling Breath: Variations

Come into Sitting Mountain, allowing your eyes to close or softening your gaze. Start with your natural breath, inhaling and exhaling gently through your nose for several breaths. Allow your breath to slow and deepen into your belly. Now choose one of the variations below that works for you in the present moment—or create one of your own.

A. Curling the tongue (Sitali): Form your lips into an O shape. Curl your tongue lengthwise and project it out of your mouth (about three-quarters of an inch). Inhale deeply through your curled tongue and into your mouth as if drinking through a straw, making a light hissing sound. (See "Cooling Breath with Sitali" option A photo.)

"Joy is hidden in the breath."

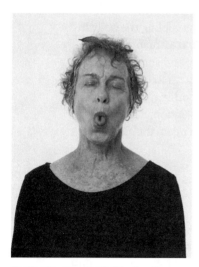

Cooling Breath with Sitali (option A)

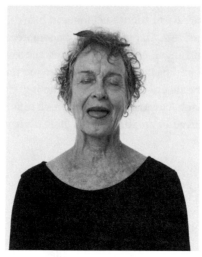

Cooling Breath with Sitkari (option B)

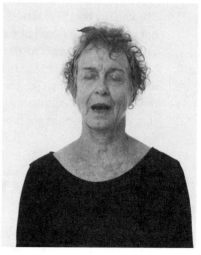

Cooling Breath with tongue on roof of mouth (option C)

B. Placing the tongue on the lower lip (Sitkari): Open your mouth slightly. Keeping the muscles of your tongue soft, protrude the tip of your tongue to rest on your lower lip. Raise the corners of your mouth slightly (with a hint of a smile). Inhale slowly over the surface of your tongue to make a soft hissing sound. (See "Cooling Breath with Sitkari" option B photo.)

C. Placing the tongue on the roof of the mouth: Open your mouth slightly. Lightly rest the tip of your tongue against the roof of your mouth behind your upper teeth, relaxing your jaw and lips. Raise the corners of your mouth slightly (with just a hint of a smile, as in option B). Inhale slowly through your mouth, allowing your breath to make a gentle hissing sound. (See "Cooling Breath with tongue on roof of mouth" option C photo.)

In all variations, after the inhale, withdraw your tongue and close your mouth. Then hold your breath briefly (optional) and relax before exhaling through your nostrils. Focus your attention on the moist cooling sensation of your breath as your abdomen and lower ribs expand on the inhale.

Tips: If rolling the tongue like a taco isn't available, just rest it on the lower lip or touch the tip to the roof of the mouth behind the front teeth for the same cooling effect.

Duration: Continue for several rounds or for two to three minutes, and then return to diaphragmatic breathing for several more breaths. If you wish to build up this practice, alternate the cooling breath for two to three minutes with diaphragmatic breathing, gradually working up to a ten-minute practice (as available). At the end of the practice, release and return to your natural breath.

Humming Bee Breath (Bhramari Pranayama)

The Humming Bee Breath is said to calm the nervous system and soothe the mind. It involves making a light humming sound on the exhale while closing off some external senses. Its Sanskrit name, *bhramari*, comes from a word meaning "humming black bee," and the practice is named after a black bee in India, whose buzzing noise is similar to the beelike sound created in the practice.

HUMMING BEE BREATH
How It Works

With the Humming Bee Breath, we block the external senses of sight and sound, which enhances the vibrations of the humming noise as it resonates through our body-mind. This physical vibration of sound can help balance the nervous system; it can also help bring us into the present moment, supporting mindful awareness. It is a gentle way of introducing sound into a yoga practice, perhaps encouraging an interest in chanting or mantras, other classic yoga techniques that use sound (see chapter 12).

When doing this breath practice, inhale naturally and exhale the hum for as long as is comfortable, keeping the buzzing sound at a moderate volume and the hum light. Humming helps to elongate the exhale, which increases its calming effect. For those with breathing challenges, hum to the natural length of your exhale or simply use visualizations (option A below) to access the benefits of this breathing practice.

Humming Bee Breath: Variations

Come into Sitting Mountain, allowing your eyes to close or softening your gaze, and touch your lips together lightly. Start with your natural breath, inhaling and exhaling gently through your nose for several breaths. Allow your breath to slow and deepen into your belly. Now choose one of the variations below that works for you in the present moment—or create one of your own.

A. Using visualization: Relax your hands on your lap and touch your lips together lightly. To help maintain focus, turn your attention inward to block all external sights and sounds. Bring an image to mind, perhaps picture yourself sitting in a garden, seeing and hearing bumble bees buzzing around colorful flowers, or come up with your own visualization. Inhale with a natural breath, then hum the exhale.

B. Closing the ears: Push your index fingers or thumbs on the small flaps that cover the opening of each ear to block out all external sounds. Inhale with a natural breath, then hum the exhale.

C. Sealing off the senses (Shanmukhi Mudra): Bring the tips of your little fingers together underneath your mouth and the tips of your ring fingers together above your mouth to help your lips stay gently closed. Let your middle fingers rest lightly on either side of your nose, keeping your nostrils open to allow your breath to flow. Put your index fingers softly on top of your shut eyelids. Place your thumbs on the small flaps covering the openings of your ears and press in to block external sounds. Inhale with a natural breath, then hum the exhale. (See "Humming Bee Breath with Shanmukhi Mudra" photo.)

In all variations, relax the muscles of your face and jaw, let your lower teeth drop down slightly to separate from your upper teeth, and place your tongue on the roof of your mouth. Focus your attention on the effects of humming on your body-mind.

Tips: If you wish to further explore the physical sensations of vibration in your body-mind, place your hands on various parts of your body as available—such as your abdomen, your chest, the outside of your throat or jaw, the top of your head—at the beginning or end of a Humming Bee Breath practice. It can be interesting and fun to move your hands around to different body parts (or visualize this) to find out where the vibration may be enhanced, subdued, or even absent.

Duration: Continue to inhale naturally through your nose and hum the exhale for one to three minutes, building up gradually to fifteen minutes (as available). At the end of the practice, release and return to your natural breath, feeling the vibration of the whole body-mind.

*"Sound has the power to heal—opening the breath,
opening the body, opening the mind, opening the heart."*

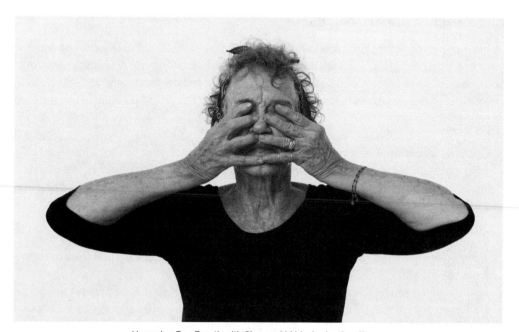

Humming Bee Breath with Shanmukhi Mudra (option C)

Three-Part Breath (Dirgha Pranayama)

Three-Part Breath is said to cultivate deep-breathing awareness, increase lung capacity, and generate calm in the body-mind. It involves bringing attention to three areas where the breath is most apparent (besides the nostrils): (1) the collarbones, chest, and upper lungs; (2) the rib cage, lower lungs, and upper abdomen; and (3) the diaphragm and lower abdomen. The word *dirgha* means "long" in Sanskrit, which expresses how this breathing practice encourages a lengthening of the inhale, the exhale, or both. It can also be translated as "deep," and the practice is sometimes referred to as "the complete breath," emphasizing further qualities fostered by the Three-Part Breath.

THREE-PART BREATH
How It Works

Dirgha pranayama is one of the most effective practices for breathing deeper and slower, which has many wellness benefits, including making fuller use of the lungs; stretching the intercostals and other muscles of the rib cage, chest, and abdomen; relaxing the whole body-mind; and relieving stress. Deep breathing is also known as diaphragmatic, abdominal, or belly breathing. These terms may be used interchangeably.

Traditionally with this technique, the breath is invited to expand into the belly first, starting low in the abdomen, climbing up into the rib cage, then rising into the chest, all during one inhale. The direction is reversed on the exhale, beginning with the chest, then the rib cage, and then the belly (see option C). As this pattern may not be available to beginners and others, we have developed two further options. In option A, breath awareness starts with the chest first instead of the abdomen, with a full round of breath (inhale, exhale) taken at each body area before moving to the next area. In option B, the breath is inhaled in three parts as in option C, followed by one smooth, continuous, and long exhale, which increases the calming effect of this breath practice.

With Three-Part Breath, the breath is sipped (on the inbreath and/or the outbreath) in three equal lengths at each body area, with the goal of keeping the breath steady and even. To help create a steady and even breath, you can combine this technique with Victorious Breath (see page 74), using a gentle restriction of your throat muscles to increase control and concentration while following the breathing patterns outlined below. To avoid pulling, pushing, or holding your breath, start with option A, then move to option B and/or C as available, gaining further benefits from this breathing technique.

In all variations, it can be helpful to place one hand or both hands on each body area in turn to feel how your breath moves in your body, increasing mindful awareness. (See the photos illustrating the options offered for "Breathing with hands on abdomen/ribs/chest in Three-Part Breath," page 73) If use of your hands is not available, then visualizing the movement of your body and breath can be equally beneficial. Please note that we don't actually breathe into the belly—the lungs don't extend that far down! Rather, we use the breath to create an expansion in the belly as the diaphragm moves, which helps us access the benefits of slow, deep breathing.

Three-Part Breath: Variations

Come into Sitting Mountain, allowing your eyes to close or softening your gaze. Start with your natural breath, inhaling and exhaling gently through your nose for several breaths. Now choose one of the variations below that works for you in the present moment—or create your own.

A. Inhaling and exhaling at each body area: Place one or two hands on your chest or visualize doing so by simply bringing your attention there. Inhale slowly, noticing your breath as your chest rises. Exhale slowly, noticing your breath as your chest descends. Then move your hand(s) and attention to your rib cage, or visualize this. Inhale slowly, noticing your breath as your torso expands out like an accordion. Exhale slowly, noticing your torso as it releases inward. And now move your hand(s) to your lower abdomen, or visualize this. Inhale slowly, noticing your breath as your abdomen grows, as if there's a balloon inflating inside your belly. Exhale, noticing the balloon deflating and your belly relaxing. Repeat.

B. Inhaling Three-Part Breath: Place one hand on your abdomen and the other on your chest, or visualize this. Exhale deeply to empty the lungs and prepare to sip the inhale in three parts. Bringing your attention to your lower abdomen, inhale a small sip of air and allow your belly to expand. Next bring your attention to your upper abdomen and inhale another small sip of air, allowing your rib cage to expand. Now bring your attention to your chest and inhale a third small sip of air, allowing your collarbones to rise. Exhale slowly and smoothly, noticing your whole torso as it releases inward.

C. Inhaling and exhaling Three-Part Breath: Place one hand on your abdomen and the other on your chest, or visualize this. Exhale deeply to empty the lungs and prepare to sip the inhale in three parts. Bringing your attention to your lower abdomen, inhale a small sip of air and allow your belly to expand. Next bring your attention to your upper abdomen and inhale another small sip of air, allowing your rib cage to expand. Now bring your attention to your chest and inhale a third small sip of air, allowing your collarbones to rise. Slowly and steadily, exhale a small sip of air and let your chest descend first. Exhale a bit more and let your rib cage release inward. Then exhale a bit more and let your belly relax.

Tips: To help maintain a steady and even breath and aid concentration, lightly engage your throat muscles using Victorious Breath (page 74). Or come up with a visualization, such as imagining your breath filling your entire body on the inbreath and completely emptying your body on the outbreath. The photos that accompany this pranayama help illustrate the options offered.

Duration: When first practicing this technique, repeat the breath cycle three times or for one to three minutes, building up gradually to ten to twenty minutes (as available). At the end of the practice, release and return to your natural breath.

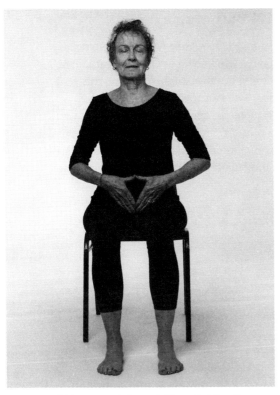

Breathing with hands on abdomen in Three-Part Breath

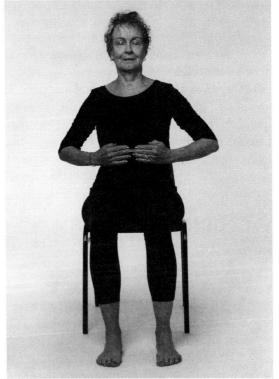

Breathing with hands on ribs in Three-Part Breath

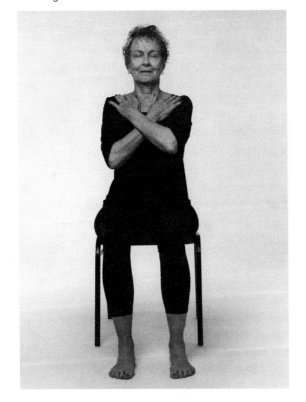

Breathing with hands on chest in Three-Part Breath

"Through breath, movement, and meditation, the body-mind becomes longer, stronger, and lighter."

Victorious Breath (Ujjayi Pranayama)

Victorious Breath is said to calm and balance the body-mind, increase oxygen in the blood, strengthen the muscles of the throat, and warm the body. Also known as Ocean Breath, it involves creating a sound like an ocean wave by tightening the throat muscles to restrict and control the flow of air in and out of the nostrils. The word *ujjayi* translates as "one who is victorious," which suggests that practicing this breathing technique can help us achieve our intention, whatever that may be: staying focused and present, synchronizing physical body movements with the movement of the breath, improving attention and concentration, calming the fluctuations of the mind, creating steadiness and balance in the body, reaching a state of meditation (*dhyana*) or even joy or bliss (*samadhi*).

VICTORIOUS BREATH

How It Works

Victorious Breath is very versatile—it is commonly used in both breathing and meditation practices, either on its own or combined with other techniques such as Three-Part Breath (see page 71) and Coherent Breathing (see page 76). It has also been a focus in some asana practices, both traditional and modern. In modern Ashtanga and Vinyasa yoga styles, this breath is often done quite vigorously, with sound that can be heard by others in the room; or it can be done gently, with just a hint of sound in one's own ears. Feel free to use it with any of the chair-asanas in chapter 9 and meditation practices in chapter 10.

With Victorious Breath, the inhale and exhale can be the same length (1:1 ratio), which balances the nervous system, or the inhale can be followed by a longer exhale (1:2 ratio), which produces calm. In both instances, the goal is to maintain a smooth and regular rhythm. For beginners and those who experience breathlessness, start with a ratio of 2:2 (inhale for a count of two, exhale for a count of two) or 2:4 (inhale for a count of two, exhale for a count of four). Or even ratios 1:1 or 1:2 are fine!

When first learning this technique, students often wonder if they are doing it correctly, and some even experience a sore throat. To aid learning and to allow your throat muscles to get used to the practice, see the steps outlined below (option A). Be patient as you learn, starting with options A and B to avoid pulling, pushing, or holding your breath, then move to option C if available, gaining further benefits from this breathing technique. A word of caution: Victorious Breath builds heat in the body and activates the throat. If you are experiencing any respiratory symptoms, such as inflammation, coughing, or wheezing, you may prefer to simply visualize ocean waves flowing in and out with the natural breath.

Victorious Breath: Variations

Come into Sitting Mountain, allowing your eyes to close or softening your gaze. Start with your natural breath, inhaling and exhaling gently through your nose for several breaths. Allow your breath to slow and deepen into your belly. Now choose one of the variations below that works for you in the present moment—or create one of your own.

A. Creating sound with Victorious Breath: Bring one palm up in front of your face, as if you are looking into a hand mirror. Inhale slowly through your nose. Then open your mouth and breathe out warm air onto your palm, as if you are fogging up the imaginary hand mirror, and make a long "haaa" sound aloud. Inhale and exhale in this way one or two more times. Inhale slowly again, and on the next exhale, keeping your mouth closed, breathe out as if the "haaa" sound is now coming out of your throat. If you wish, place a finger or two on the front of your throat to feel the muscles vibrating or contracting as you breathe the sound out. (See photo "Feeling muscle contraction in throat in Victorious Breath.")

B. Exhaling Victorious Breath: Draw your breath in slowly through your nose. Exhale through your nose while contracting the muscles in the back of your throat and creating either a soft snore-like sound or the sound of an ocean wave as your breath passes through your windpipe.

C. Inhaling and exhaling Victorious Breath: Inhale slowly through your nose while contracting the muscles in the back of your throat, creating the sound of either a soft snore or an ocean wave. Repeat on the exhale.

In all variations, keep the sound soft and gentle, or to create more energy or warmth, make the sound louder and perhaps noticeable enough so that someone sitting next to you can hear it. Choose a rhythm that suits you in the present moment: equal inhales and exhales (1:1 ratio) or longer exhales (1:2 ratio). As you engage Victorious Breath, allow your abdomen to move out and in as in the Three-Part Breath, expanding with the inhalation and contracting with the exhalation.

Tips: To help maintain a steady rhythm and aid concentration, imagine your breath moving in and out with the tide across a sandy or stony beach, or come up with your own visualization.

Duration: Begin with a few rounds or practice for one to three minutes, building up gradually to ten to twenty minutes (as available). At the end of the practice, release and return to your natural breath.

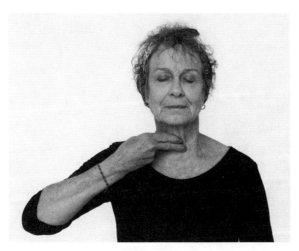

"Becoming absorbed in the sound and movement of our own breath brings us into the present moment."

Feeling muscle contraction in throat in Victorious Breath

Coherent Breathing

Coherent Breathing is a slow breathing technique that is said to enhance respiratory, circulatory, and neurological health and balance all the systems of the body-mind. Also known as resonant breathing, it involves inhaling and exhaling at a rate of five or six breaths per minute, and there are no pauses between the breaths. Research has shown that Coherent Breathing can optimize heart rate variability (HRV).[10] HRV is a key measure of cardiovascular health. Other benefits associated with Coherent Breathing include greater flexibility in the nervous system and better oxygenation of the body.

COHERENT BREATHING
How It Works

With Coherent Breathing, the inhale and exhale are the same length, and the goal is to make the breath smooth, even, and continuous, with no pauses between the breaths. If you're new to this practice or are experiencing any signs of breathlessness, start with a count of 2:2—that is, inhale for a count of two, exhale for a count of two, with each count lasting one second. This facilitates keeping your breath smooth and helps you avoid pulling, pushing, or holding your breath. Then begin to build up, as available, to a count of 5:5 or 6:6—breathing in for five or six seconds, breathing out for five or six seconds, which equates to five or six breaths per minute—to gain maximum benefit from this breathing technique. If you feel agitated at any point or your breath becomes jagged, return to a count that feels smooth and even.

To help maintain a slow, smooth, and even breath, combine Coherent Breathing with Victorious Breath (see page 74), using a gentle restriction of your throat muscles to increase control and attention while following the breathing pattern outlined below. To help maintain the rhythm, you can count your breaths mentally to yourself or enlist an external source to assist. For example, a yoga teacher or other person can count aloud for you. Or listen to the sound of a chime or the beat of a metronome, set to the desired ratio, using a tally counter (available as a separate device or downloaded as an app on your cell phone or other electronic device).

"Living in the rhythm of the breath is like living in the rhythm of a dance."

Coherent Breathing: Variations

Come into Sitting Mountain, allowing your eyes to close or softening your gaze. Start with your natural breath, inhaling and exhaling gently through your nose for several breaths. Allow your breath to slow and deepen into your belly. Now choose one of the variations below that works for you in the present moment—or create your own.

A. Coherent Breathing to a count of 2:2. Breathe in slowly, expanding your abdomen, to a count of two. Slowly breathe out, letting your abdomen relax, to a count of two.

B. Coherent Breathing to a count of 3:3 or 4:4. Breathe in slowly, expanding your abdomen, to a count of three or four. Slowly breathe out, letting your abdomen relax, to a count of three or four.

C. Coherent Breathing to a count of 5:5 or 6:6. Breathe in slowly, expanding your abdomen, to a count of five or six. Slowly breathe out, letting your abdomen relax, to a count of five or six.

Tips: To help maintain a smooth and even breath and aid concentration, lightly engage your throat muscles using Victorious Breath (see page 74). Or come up with a visualization, such as imagining your breath moving easily and continuously along a circular path, inhaling along the top half of the circle and exhaling along the bottom half of the circle, transitioning smoothly between the inhales and exhales.

Duration: Begin by practicing for one to three minutes, building up gradually to ten to twenty minutes per day (as available). At the end of the practice, release and return to your natural breath.

9

Forty Poses on the Chair

Asana is steady, comfortable posture.

—PATANJALI, *Yoga Sutras* 2:46

ASANAS—the poses or postures in yoga—provide purposeful movement that can help the body improve and/or maintain one's strength, flexibility, and coordination through all stages of life. As such, they can be considered a mindfulness activity, just like a breathing exercise or a meditation. Asanas are often the most recognizable images of yoga, and for many, these purposeful movements are a vital technique for accessing yoga's benefits.

In this chapter, we present forty poses that we have adapted to the chair, organized alphabetically. Each pose includes:

- Three "Single Chair Yoga" versions illustrating different levels of flexibility (options A, B, and C)

- Another view of option C on the chair—from the side, front, or angle

- A mat version of the pose—from which the chair options are adapted

- Step-by-step instructions

- Awareness tips for students and teachers

Also included for each pose are a number of potential physical and mental health benefits; suggestions for where to focus the eyes (*drishti*); and one or more counterposes. A counterpose brings the body back into a neutral position or stretches it in the opposite direction. Please note that Sitting Mountain is a neutral counterpose for every posture.

For an explanation of precautions in our chair-yoga approach and more details for certain conditions, see the tips for specific poses and also chapter 12 on safety. For guidance on how to build your own chair-yoga practice and tips on choosing which poses to do, see chapter 13 on building a Lakshmi Voelker Method sequence.

Let this chapter serve as a guide and a reference as you explore our chair-yoga method. While we provide detailed instructions for only three options for each pose, there are endless variations as well as the option to visualize. Once you embrace the chair-yoga practice presented in this book, you can come up with your own options, using your sat nam to safely, effectively, and skillfully adapt any pose to the chair.

How to Use Step-by-Step Instructions for Chair-Asanas

The step-by-step instructions for the poses are designed to aid coming into and out of each chair-asana safely and effectively, whether you are practicing by yourself or teaching others.

Each pose incorporates various features of our chair-yoga method, which are explained in detail in part two of this book. To make the most of these instructions and for practicing safely, it is useful to familiarize yourself with our levels of flexibility (chapter 4) and the step-by-step instructions for Sitting Mountain (chapter 5). Review our alignment principles (chapter 6) as well. For the lower body: press points in the feet (pages 55–56); leg position options (pages 52–53); and foot placement options (page 54). For the upper body: eye focus (*drishti*), especially high seam and low seam, and neck safety (pages 47–48); raising and lowering the arms (pages 48–50); and folding forward from the hips (pages 50–51).

Feel free to make an audio recording of the instructions to more easily follow the movements, choosing the levels of flexibility—options A, B, or C—that work for you in the present moment. Remember that it's fine to choose different options for your lower and upper body as well as for the left and right sides. And choosing to visualize any movement is always an option!

Tips for Practicing Asanas

Start each asana practice with Sitting Mountain, our foundational pose (see chapter 5). Be sure your chair is stable, secure, and adjusted to suit your body, using props under your feet, behind your back, or under your buttocks as needed to sit toward the front edge of the chair in good postural alignment. Spend a few moments following your natural breath before you start practicing.

For each pose or practice, ask yourself, "What is my intention? What am I trying to achieve with this pose?" Understanding your intention allows you to focus on what you want to get out of each movement, so that you gain the desired benefits while keeping safe.

Then explore different variations of the pose, starting with a basic version (such as option A) and moving into other modifications (options B or C), depending on your intention and level of flexibility. Feel free to move around on your chair and readjust to find a comfortable seat in any pose. Remember to mix and match to what suits your body-mind on the day!

To aid strength and resilience, you can hold poses in a still or a static manner in your chosen level of flexibility. How long should a pose be held? We often recommend holding a pose for three breaths; begin with one or two breaths and build up during the practice or over time as available.

For flexibility and coordination, our poses can be practiced with flowing or dynamic movements. How many times should a pose be repeated? Again, start small with one to three repetitions and increase over time as available, honoring where your body is in each particular practice.

For maximum safety, come into and out of poses slowly and deliberately, one body part at a time. Set up your lower body first to establish a stable base, then set up your upper body; do the opposite when coming out of a pose—returning your upper body first, then your lower body, to a safe neutral position—and then return to Sitting Mountain. In addition to working our physical muscles, this also helps us to be mindful and enhances our ability to pay attention.

Sometimes you can concentrate so hard when doing an asana that you hold your breath—remind yourself to keep breathing!

Tips for Teaching Asanas

To make the practice as accessible as possible, we ask students to explore different variations of a pose, starting with a basic version (such as option A or visualization) and moving into other modifications (such as options B or C), depending on the student's level of flexibility. Remind your students to mix and match to what suits their body-mind on the day.

When we guide our students, it is important that both our verbal instructions and visual demonstrations are offered mindfully—remember matrika shakti when "speaking" with voice and body. (See also the section on "Using Props and Assists" in chapter 12 on pages 215 for further helpful tips.)

Remember that any style of yoga can be adapted to the chair using our levels of flexibility— use your own sat nam, your own authentic self, to explore!

Be sure to ask for feedback from your students and listen. In our experience, we learn something new from our students every day, enhancing the gifts we receive from and give to others through our chair-yoga practice.

When coming into a chair-asana, remember to start in Sitting Mountain and find the level of flexibility that suits you on that day. When releasing a chair-asana, return to Sitting Mountain by coming back one limb and one breath at a time.

Tips for Practicing Asana on a Wheelchair and for Teaching Wheelchair Users

Although any class or sequence using our chair-yoga approach can offer safe and effective adaptations for those who use wheelchairs (wheelchairs are chairs, after all!), we provide some specific suggestions on how wheelchair users can make the most of their experience and how teachers can support their students who use wheelchairs.

All asanas, breathing practices, and meditations can be adapted to the wheelchair applying our levels of flexibility. Practicing wheelchair yoga may enhance a wheelchair user's connection and "friendship" with their wheelchair, making it more of an extension of their body. It can also improve gross motor skills, increase focus and concentration, and develop self-esteem, fostering greater harmony, strength, and flexibility.

At the start of every practice, be sure that the wheels of the chair are locked for safety. The footrests can be used, or they can be moved to the side of the wheelchair so the feet can press directly onto the ground or on props placed under the feet. Other props, such as cushions, can be used as assists for the arms and back as well. If a teacher or caregiver is to offer physical assists, then be sure that consent has been obtained beforehand, in accordance with Yoga Alliance's Code of Conduct on consent-based touch.[11] (See chapter 12 for more information.)

As with any practice utilizing our approach, begin in Sitting Mountain (see page 41, 45). In this chapter, we offer three examples on a wheelchair featuring one of our wheelchair students: Tree Pose is illustrated with three suggested levels of flexibility (see pages 164–65). Bound Angle Pose is presented with one proposed option for this asana using props (see page 86), and Dancer Pose shows how a wheelchair user might be assisted in doing this posture (see page 103). We invite students and teachers to use our levels of flexibility to find other options and variations for the poses in this chapter that work for them.

Be sure to bring your sat nam, your own creativity and authenticity, to practice wheelchair yoga using our approach and, if you teach, to your students who use wheelchairs. As Matthew Sanford, a wheelchair user and widely recognized author, yoga teacher, and pioneer in adapting yoga for people with disabilities, writes: "I've never known someone to become more at home in his or her body, in all its flaws and its grace, without becoming more compassionate to all of life."

A Note for Everyone

Our chair-yoga method has been designed to keep you safe. We encourage you to be gentle with your body as you explore chair-yoga postures. This is not about attaining perfection; rather, it is about engaging well with our bodies. If we go too fast or do too much, we may injure or distress our systems. Listen to your body and do what works at the pace that suits you.

As with any exercise or movement-based activity, it is advisable to check with your doctor first before starting a chair-yoga practice, in particular if it has been some time since you exercised regularly and/or you have health issues, including any inflammation or any symptoms that concern you. "When in doubt, check it out."[12]

BOAT POSE

(Navasana)

Begin in Sitting Mountain. Turn and face the right side of the chair and reestablish Sitting Mountain. Keep your right buttock on the chair; your left buttock may extend off the chair as needed, keeping both sit bones on the chair.

LOWER BODY: Come onto the balls of your feet and hinge back from your hips. Engaging the muscles of your abdomen, buttocks, and thighs, choose to either:

A. Stay in that position;
B. Lift your left leg, with your knee bent or straight; or
C. Lift both legs, with knees bent or straight.

Note: For extra support, hold on to the chair seat as you explore the different options for setting up your lower body.

UPPER BODY: Keeping your arms shoulder-width apart, turn your palms to face each other and either:

A. Rest the outsides of your hands on your thighs, elbows bent and in close to your body;
B. Lift your hands to chest height, keeping your elbows bent; or
C. Extend your arms straight out parallel to the ground, as available.

Putting it all together: As you hinge back from your hips, draw your shoulders back and down, lengthening your torso and spine. Lift your sternum and engage your upper-body muscles, stretching your hands and arms, as available, or visualizing them stretching. Gaze forward or up to the high seam. With option B for the lower body, repeat with your right leg. To come out of the pose, return to Sitting Mountain on the right side of the chair and then move to the front of the chair into Sitting Mountain.

Tips: If you're using a chair with arms, begin in Sitting Mountain facing forward. Come onto the ball of one foot and bring it back toward the chair as far as available, then hinge back from your hips; follow the steps above, beginning with your lower body.

If you are pregnant or are menstruating, you may want to skip Boat Pose if it causes discomfort, or choose more basic options, or simply visualize the pose from Sitting Mountain.

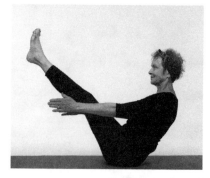

Boat Pose, on the mat

BENEFITS: PHYSICAL
- Improves balance and coordination
- Builds core strength
- Strengthens legs, groin, hips, abdomen, and arms
- Lengthens spine and neck
- Opens chest, shoulders, and throat
- Improves posture
- Enhances digestion and circulation

BENEFIT: MENTAL
- Develops focus and concentration

EYE FOCUS
- Forward
- High seam

COUNTERPOSES
- Sitting Mountain
- Knee-to-Chest Pose

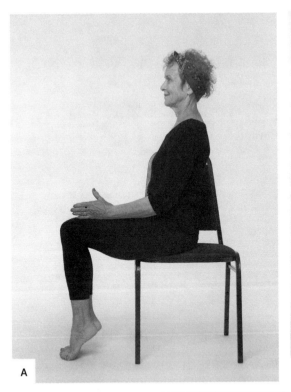

A

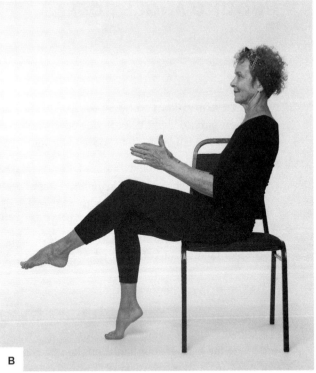

B

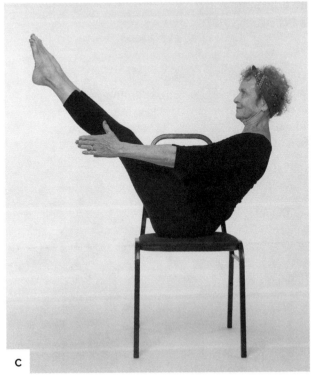

C

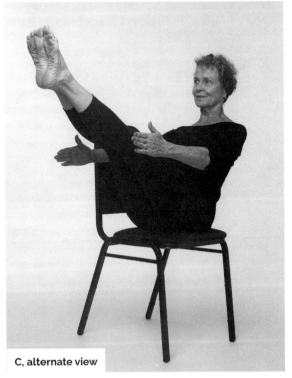

C, alternate view

BOUND ANGLE POSE

(Baddha Konasana)

Begin in Sitting Mountain.

LOWER BODY: Turn both feet out so that they are resting on their outer edges, little-toe side down, allowing your hips and knees to fall open, and choose to either:

A. Stay in that position, with your feet hip-width apart;

B. Stay in that position and bring the soles of your feet to face each other, feet in line with your navel; or

C. Use props—place one or two blocks under each foot to raise your turned-out feet as high as available with your soles facing each other.

UPPER BODY: Choose to either:

A. Rest the outside (little finger side) of your hands on your thighs, opening your palms;

B. Rest the back of your hands on the inside of your thighs and open your palms; or

C. Raise your hands to abdomen or chest height, bringing the outside edges of your hands together, and open your palms.

Putting it all together: Once you find your level of flexibility, draw your shoulders back and down, lengthening your torso and spine. Lift your sternum as you continue to open your hips and the palms of your hands. Gaze forward or down to the low seam. Come out of the pose and return to Sitting Mountain.

Tips: Opening the knees encourages the hips and inner thighs to open and stretch, as well as the soles of the feet. Also shown here is a further option on a wheelchair using props.

This pose is also known as Butterfly Pose and Cobbler's Pose.

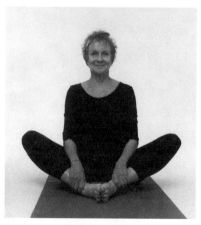

Bound Angle Pose, on the mat

BENEFITS: PHYSICAL
- Stretches thighs, groin, and hips
- Opens chest
- Lengthens spine
- Stimulates circulation

BENEFIT: MENTAL
- Reduces stress

EYE FOCUS
- Forward
- Low seam

COUNTERPOSE
- Sitting Mountain

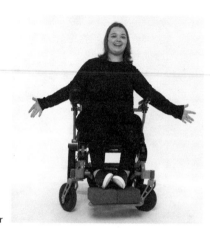

Bound Angle Pose, on a wheelchair

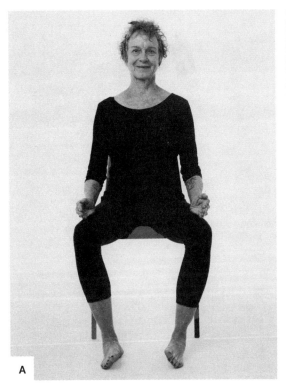

A

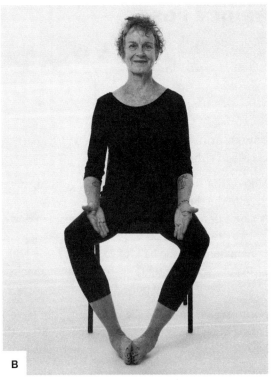

B

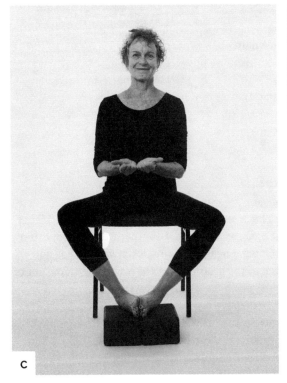

C

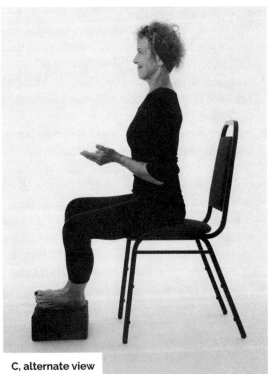

C, alternate view

BRIDGE POSE

(Setu Bandha Sarvangasana/
Setu Bandhasana)

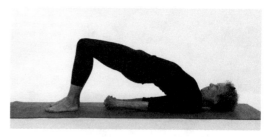

Bridge Pose, on the mat

Begin in Sitting Mountain.

LOWER BODY: With your legs hip-width apart, choose to either:

A. Keep the soles of your feet on the ground, pushing down onto the three press points;

B. Come onto the balls of both feet, pushing down onto the two press points; or

C. Remaining on the balls of your feet, move both feet back toward the chair up to six inches, as available, and push down onto the two press points.

Note: An alternative for the lower body is to leave your legs in Sitting Mountain and engage the press points in the *heels* of both feet instead of the press points in the balls of your feet.

UPPER BODY: With your arms by your sides, choose to either:

A. Keep them by your sides, elbows bent, and hold the chair seat on either side;

B. Bring your hands behind your back and hold on to the back of the chair seat, with your fingers pointing backward; or

C. Bring your hands behind your back, interlace your fingers, and straighten your arms, as available.

Putting it all together: Once you find your level of flexibility, push down onto the press points in your feet and engage your leg and abdominal muscles. Draw your shoulders back and down, bringing your shoulder blades in toward each other; lift your sternum and arch your back, as available. Lengthen your tailbone and extend your pelvis forward toward your knees, as available. Engage the muscles of your hands and arms, tuck your chin toward your chest, and gaze down at the ground or at the low seam. Come out of the pose and return to Sitting Mountain.

Tips: As a backbend, Bridge Pose can help improve your posture as well as your mood, energizing the body and the mind. You can use similar instructions and modify further for backbends such as Bow Pose (Dhanurasana) and Upward Bow/Wheel Pose (Urdhva Dhanurasana). For those with lower-back or sacral issues: if you feel a pinch, go back an inch.

BENEFITS: PHYSICAL
- Increases strength and flexibility in spine, shoulders, and hands
- Opens hips, psoas, abdomen, chest, and shoulders
- Builds lung capacity
- Strengthens legs and feet
- Aids digestion
- Relieves backache and menstrual symptoms

BENEFITS: MENTAL
- Alleviates stress and fatigue
- Lifts mood

EYE FOCUS
- Ground
- Low seam

COUNTERPOSES
- Forward Fold
- Knee-to-Chest Pose
- Spinal Twist

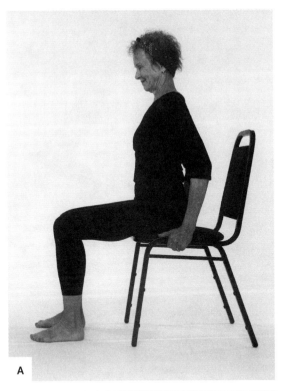

A

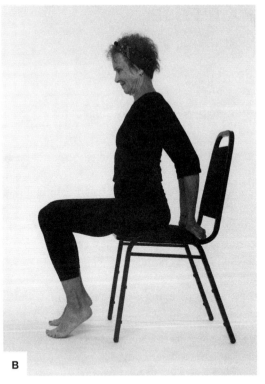

B

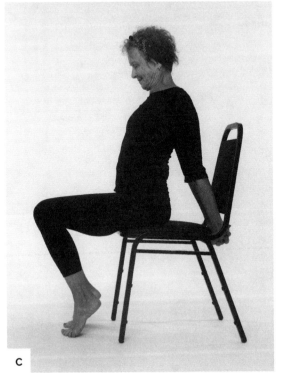

C

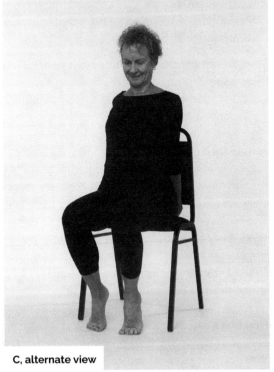

C, alternate view

CHAIR POSE

(Utkatasana)

Begin in Sitting Mountain.

LOWER BODY: With your legs hip-width apart, choose to either:

A. Keep the soles of your feet on the ground, pushing down onto the three press points;
B. Come onto the balls of both feet, pushing down onto the two press points; or
C. Remaining on the balls of your feet, move both feet back toward the chair up to six inches, as available, and push down onto the two press points.

UPPER BODY: Keeping your arms shoulder-width apart, turn your palms to face each other. Choose to either:

A. Rest the outside of your hands on your thighs, elbows bent and in close to your body;
B. Keeping your elbows bent, lift your hands to chest or shoulder height; or
C. Straighten your elbows and extend your arms as fully and as high as available.

Note: Remember that you can bring your arms anywhere between resting on your thighs to lifting them fully extended overhead next to your ears, depending on what works for you on the day.

Putting it all together: Once you find your level of flexibility, engage your leg and abdominal muscles, pushing down onto the two press points in your feet. Lengthen your torso and hinge forward at your hips, as available. Draw your shoulders back and down, lift your sternum, and engage your upper-body muscles, stretching your hands and arms out or up as far as available (or visualize the movement). Gaze forward or up to the high seam. Come out of the pose and return to Sitting Mountain.

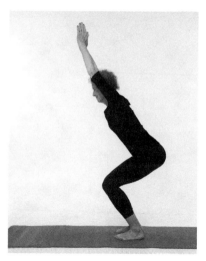

Chair Pose, on the mat

BENEFITS: PHYSICAL
- Strengthens feet, ankles, calves, knees, thighs, and buttocks
- Lengthens torso, spine, arms, and hands
- Increases abdominal and core muscle strength
- Stimulates digestion and circulation
- Improves balance

BENEFITS: MENTAL
- Develops concentration and attention
- Builds confidence

EYE FOCUS
- Forward
- High seam

COUNTERPOSE
- Sitting Mountain

Tips: Chair Pose encourages stability and balance in body and mind. If you need to make space for the belly, you can widen your legs into a V-shaped or L-shaped position. If you are lifting and raising your arms overhead, remember to soften and relax your shoulders to avoid strain. If you feel faint, lightheaded, or dizzy when raising your arms, keep your head level, looking forward with your eyes and not up.

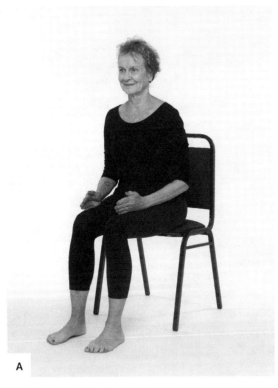

A

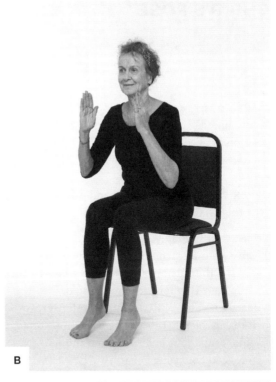

B

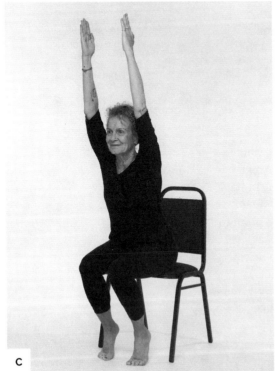

C

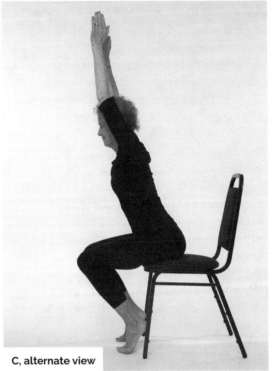

C, alternate view

CHILD'S POSE

(Balasana)

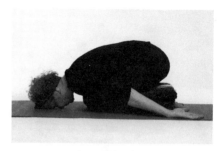

Child's Pose, on the mat

Begin in Sitting Mountain.

LOWER BODY: Keeping your legs and feet in Sitting Mountain, take care to come into V-shaped or L-shaped leg position as needed, adding enough space between your legs for your belly to rest comfortably.

UPPER BODY: Hinge forward and place your elbows onto your thighs. Choose to either:

A. Rest your head in your hands;
B. Cross your forearms, gently resting or clasping your hands around the outside of your elbows; lower your head and drop your chin toward your chest; or
C. Place a soft prop or two onto your lap; cross your forearms, gently resting them on your prop(s); drop your chin, drape your body over your prop(s), and lower your forehead onto your forearms.

Putting it all together: Child's Pose should feel comfortable and easeful. If you choose option C, make sure you've stacked enough props to support your upper body and to comfortably rest your head on your forearms. Lower your gaze or close your eyes. Add either Victorious Breath or Coherent Breathing if that feels relaxing to you. Come out of the pose and return to Sitting Mountain.

Tips: Props can be anything that allows you to release your head and neck comfortably. The support of your torso and spine provided by props also allows you to relax safely in this forward-fold posture, in case of any bone loss or sinus challenges. If you feel faint, lightheaded, or dizzy, use props to keep your head above your heart, moving into whatever level of flexibility feels doable and visualizing the rest. We recommend using a bolster or two, a few blankets, a firm pillow or two, or even a large exercise ball to drape your body over. You may discover other soft props that work better for you.

BENEFITS: PHYSICAL
- Stretches and lengthens spine
- Relaxes muscles of front body
- Massages internal organs
- Stimulates digestion and circulation
- May ease head, neck, and chest challenges and insomnia

BENEFITS: MENTAL
- Calms the mind
- Reduces fatigue and stress

EYE FOCUS
- Downward
- Eyes closed or soft

COUNTERPOSES
- Sitting Mountain
- Backbends

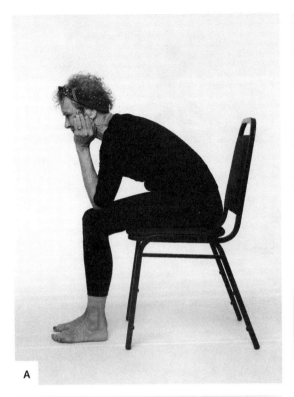

A

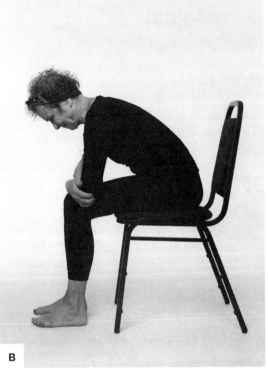

B

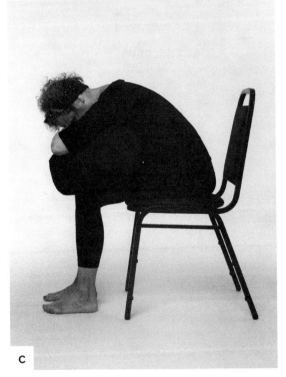

C

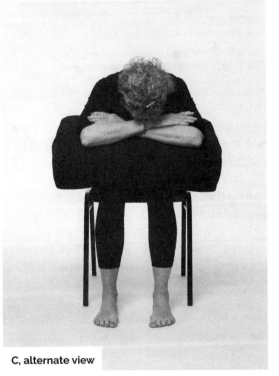

C, alternate view

COBRA POSE

(Bhujangasana)

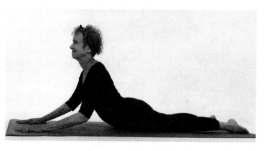

Cobra Pose, on the mat

Begin in Sitting Mountain.

LOWER BODY: Come onto the balls of both feet, pushing down onto the two press points. Choose to either:

A. Stay in that position;
B. Remaining on the balls of your feet, move both feet back a few inches toward the chair; or
C. Remaining on the balls of your feet, move both feet back even farther up to six inches, as available.

UPPER BODY: Place your hands on your thighs, spreading your fingers wide, as available, and bend your elbows in close to your body. Choose to either:

A. Flex your hands up at your wrists, keeping the heels of your hands on your thighs;
B. Raise your flexed hands up to chest height, palms facing out, and elbows in close to your body; or
C. Raise your hands up to shoulder or head height, palms facing out, with elbows in right angles and forearms slightly forward in front of your body.

Note: An alternative for option C is to bring your raised hands directly in front of or in line with your shoulders, palms facing out, and draw your elbows in close to your body for a variation called Baby (or Half) Cobra Pose (Ardha Bhujangasana).

BENEFITS: PHYSICAL
- Lengthens and strengthens spine
- Stretches chest, shoulders, and abdomen
- Firms buttocks
- Builds strength in arms and wrists
- Builds lung capacity
- Stimulates digestion and circulation

BENEFITS: MENTAL
- Relieves stress and fatigue
- Lifts mood

EYE FOCUS
- Forward
- High seam

COUNTERPOSES
- Downward-Facing Dog
- Forward Fold

Putting it all together: Once you find your level of flexibility, engage your thigh and abdominal muscles by pushing down onto the two press points in your feet. Engage your upper-body muscles by lengthening your torso, lifting your sternum and chin slightly, and bringing your shoulder blades together. Keep your elbows slightly forward in right angles, as available. Hinge back slightly, stretching your fingers and pushing your palms and forearms against an imaginary wall in front of you. Gaze forward or up to the high seam. Come out of the pose and return to Sitting Mountain.

Tips: A key backbend in Sun Salutations, Cobra Pose helps improve posture as well as mood. Use the same instructions for a deeper backbend on the mat or create further modifications using our chair-yoga method. If you have a headache or wrist challenges, you can still gain benefit by visualizing the movements.

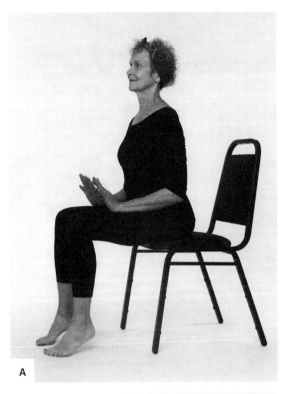

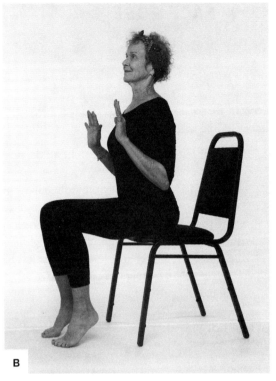

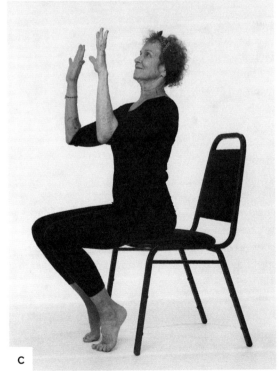

A

B

C

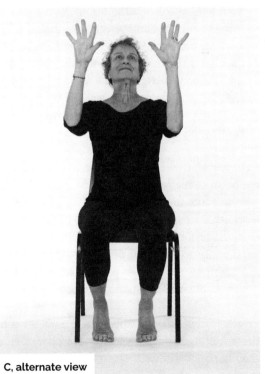

C, alternate view

COW FACE POSE
(Gomukhasana)

Begin in Sitting Mountain.

LOWER BODY: Bring both legs and feet together, with your knees in line with your navel. Choose to either:

A. Cross your left ankle over your right ankle, resting on the outer edges of your feet;

B. Position a block at its lower or middle height, just in front of the right chair leg; cross your left leg over your right, resting the outside of your left foot on the block; or

C. Position the block on its highest level, slightly away from the right front chair leg; cross your left leg over your right thigh, resting the outside edge of your left foot on the block.

UPPER BODY: With your torso facing forward, choose to either:

A. Bring your right hand onto your right shoulder and place your left hand on your left hip;

B. Bring your right hand behind your head and place the back of your left hand on your lower back; or

C. Raise your right arm up toward the ceiling, palm facing back; bend your right elbow and extend the palm of your right hand down your spine; slide the back of your left hand up your spine, clasping the fingers of both hands together, as available.

Putting it all together: Once you find your level of flexibility, begin to engage the muscles from the outside edges of your feet into the core of your pelvis. Lift your sternum and lengthen your spine, stretching the muscles in your chest, shoulders, and arms. To keep your head from tilting forward, dip your chin slightly and gently press the back of your head into your right hand or arm, or visualize doing this. Continue to stretch through the lower right side of your body as you engage the muscles in the lower left side of your body. Gaze forward or down to the low seam. Return to Sitting Mountain and repeat on the other side.

Tip: Instead of clasping your fingers together behind your back, you can hold one end of a strap, tie, or belt in each hand and tug it in opposite directions to gain a deeper stretch in your chest, shoulders, and arms.

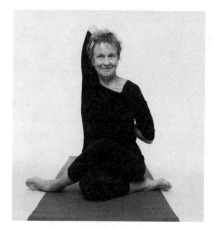

Cow Face Pose, on the mat

BENEFITS: PHYSICAL
- Opens chest, ribs, shoulders, arms, and thighs
- Increases knee flexibility and lubricates knee joint
- Lengthens spine
- Improves digestion and respiration

BENEFITS: MENTAL
- Develops focus
- Reduces stress

EYE FOCUS
- Forward
- Low seam

COUNTERPOSE
- Sitting Mountain

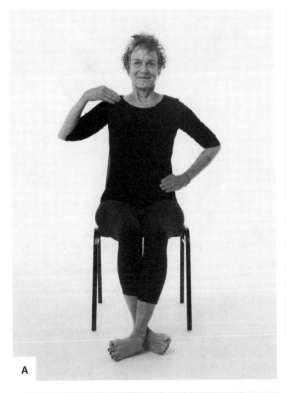

A

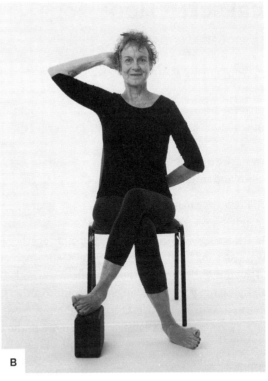

B

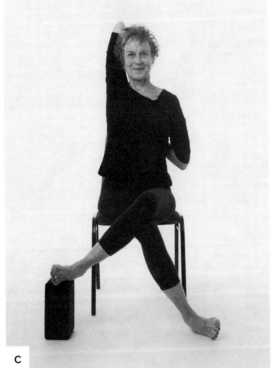

C

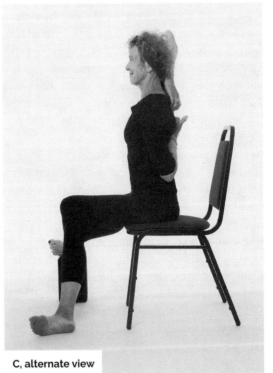

C, alternate view

CRESCENT MOON POSE

(Indudalasana)

Start in Sitting Mountain.

LOWER BODY: Keep your legs in Sitting Mountain, pushing down onto the three press points in your feet.

UPPER BODY: Bring your palms together in front of your chest and interlace your fingers. Choose to either:

A. Keep your hands at chest height and lean slightly to the left side;

B. Releasing your index fingers to point together upward, raise your hands just above your head, elbows bent, and lean slightly more to the left side; or

C. Releasing your index fingers to point together upward, reach your hands overhead, straightening your arms next to your ears as available, and lean more to the left side.

Putting it all together: Once you find your level of flexibility, engage your thigh and abdominal muscles. Lift the crown of your head toward the ceiling to lengthen your spine and the back of your neck as you relax your shoulders back and down. Lift your sternum and begin to extend and lengthen your torso to the left, pushing down onto the three press points in your feet and drawing your right shoulder back. Gaze forward or down to the low seam. Return to Sitting Mountain and repeat on the other side.

Tips: Once you set up your Crescent Moon Pose, rock from side to side in a tick-tock fashion to dynamically warm up the spine and body before holding and breathing on each side. To cultivate balance, lift the heel and come up on the toes opposite the tilt. If you are lifting and raising your arms overhead, remember to soften and relax your shoulders to avoid strain. If you feel faint, lightheaded, or dizzy when raising your arms, keep your head level, looking forward with your eyes and not up. This posture is also known as Half Moon Pose (Ardha Chandrasana) in Kripalu yoga, Bikram yoga, and other yoga styles.

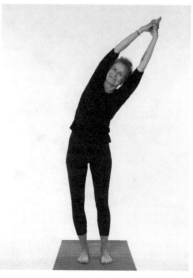
Cresent Moon Pose, on the mat

BENEFITS: PHYSICAL
- Aligns spine and improves posture
- Expands and opens chest
- Stretches arms and side body
- Tones abdominal and buttock muscles
- Strengthens arches of the feet, ankles, knees, and legs
- Stimulates circulation
- Increases lung capacity

BENEFITS: MENTAL
- Develops attention and motivation
- Improves concentration and focus
- Relieves stress

EYE FOCUS
- Forward
- Low seam

COUNTERPOSE
- Crescent Moon Pose to opposite side

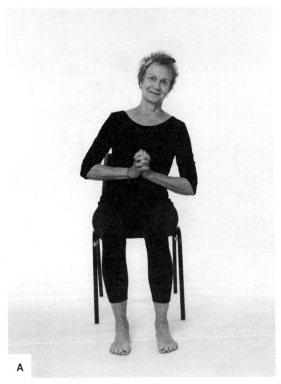

A

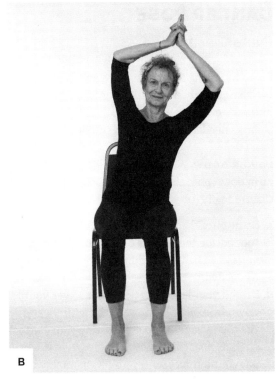

B

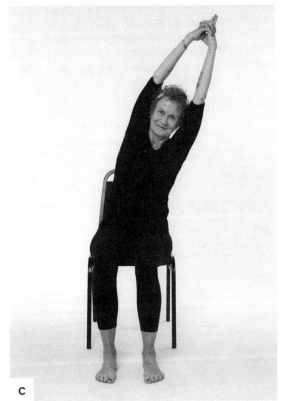

C

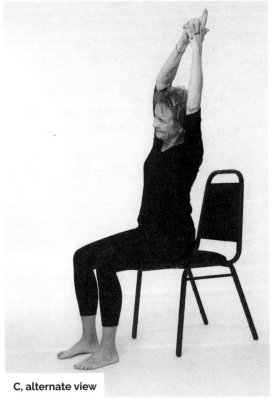

C, alternate view

DANCER POSE

(Natarajasana)

Begin in Sitting Mountain. Turn and face the right side of the chair and reestablish Sitting Mountain. Keep your right buttock on the chair; your left buttock may extend off the chair as needed, keeping both sit bones on the chair.

LOWER BODY: With your right leg in Sitting Mountain, push down onto the three press points in your right foot. Choose to either:

A. Come onto the ball of your left foot, positioning your left foot beside the outside of the front left chair leg, keeping your knee bent and adjusting your buttocks on the chair as needed;

B. Extend your left leg back farther, lower your left knee down from your hip toward the ground, and come onto the top of your left foot, adjusting your buttocks on the chair as needed; or

C. Lift your left foot with your left hand, bringing your left heel and calf toward your hamstrings and adjusting your buttocks on the chair as needed.

Note: An alternative for the extended leg in option B is to come onto the ball of your foot instead of the top and push down onto the two press points.

UPPER BODY: Keeping your arms shoulder-width apart, turn your palms to face each other. Choose to either:

A. Rest the palm of your left hand on your left thigh. Place the outside of your right hand on your right thigh, palm facing inward;

B. Extend your left arm down the left side of your body, palm facing inward. Bend your right elbow as you lift your hand up to shoulder or head height, palm facing inward; or

C. Take hold of your left foot or ankle with your left hand, pulling your heel toward your body, as available; straighten your right arm and reach overhead, as available, palm facing inward.

(CONTINUED ON NEXT SPREAD)

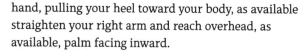

Dancer Pose, on the mat

BENEFITS: PHYSICAL
- Improves balance and coordination
- Strengthens arches, legs, and abdomen
- Stretches feet, thighs, and back
- Opens hips and psoas muscles
- Expands chest and shoulders
- Tones arms
- Improves digestion

BENEFITS: MENTAL
- Develops poise and concentration
- Relieves stress
- Calms the mind

EYE FOCUS
- Forward
- Low seam
- High seam

COUNTERPOSE
- Sitting Mountain

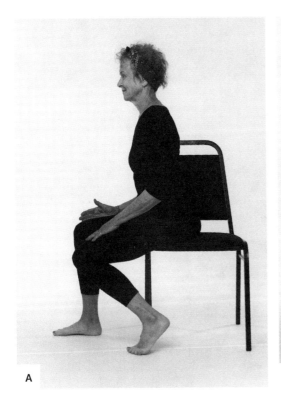

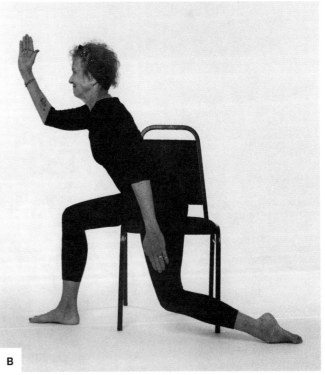

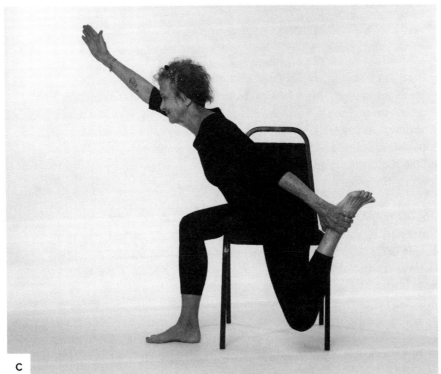

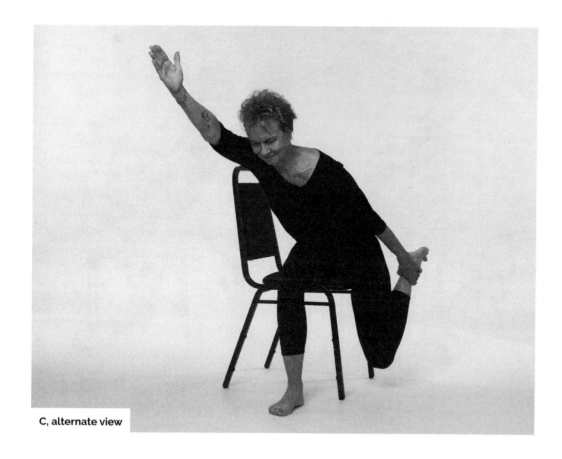

C, alternate view

Putting it all together: Once you find your level of flexibility, engage your leg muscles from your feet up into the core of your pelvis. Hinge forward from your hips, lifting the crown of your head toward the ceiling to lengthen your spine and the back of your neck, as you relax your shoulders back and down. As available, stretch or visualize this dynamic stretch through your hands and arms. Gaze forward or down to the low seam. To come out of the pose, return to Sitting Mountain on the right side of the chair and then move to the front of the chair into Sitting Mountain. Repeat on the other side.

Tips: For option C in the lower and upper body, be sure your chair is stable and you feel balanced and steady before lifting your foot off the ground. Placing a block under the knee of your raised leg can provide extra support. When you feel balanced and steady, another option for your gaze is to look up at the thumb of the raised hand or at the high seam. If you're using a chair with arms, stay in Sitting Mountain, facing forward; come onto the ball of one foot and bring it back toward the chair as far as available; then hinge forward and raise your opposite arm in front as high as available. Also shown here is an assisted option on a wheelchair. If you are lifting and raising an arm overhead, remember to soften and relax your shoulder to avoid strain. If you feel faint, lightheaded, or dizzy when raising an arm, keep your head level, looking forward with your eyes and not up.

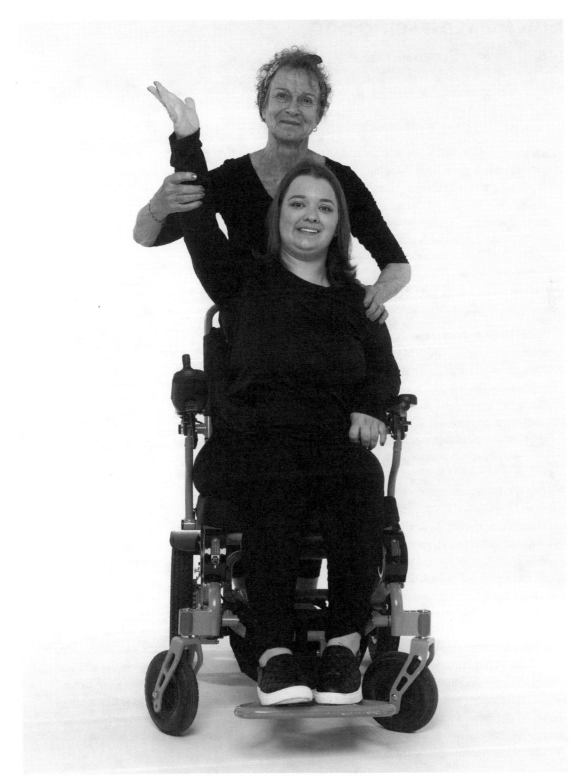

Assisted Dancer Pose, on a wheelchair

DOWNWARD-FACING DOG

(Adho Mukha Shvanasana)

Begin in Sitting Mountain.

LOWER BODY: Choose to either:

A. Keep your legs in Sitting Mountain and lift your toes;
B. Extend your legs forward, keeping your knees bent and coming up onto your heels with your feet flexed at the ankles; or
C. Extend your legs farther forward, straightening your knees as available and coming up onto your heels with your feet flexed at the ankles.

UPPER BODY: Keeping your arms shoulder-width apart, spread your fingers wide. Choose to either:

A. Place the heels of your hands on your thighs, elbows in toward your waist, and flex your hands at the wrists;
B. Lift your arms up and extend them forward at abdomen or chest height, keeping your hands flexed and your elbows either bent or straightened; or
C. Lift your arms, extending them forward and up next to your ears, as available, keeping your hands flexed and your elbows either bent or straightened.

Putting it all together: Once you find your level of flexibility, begin to hinge forward at the hips, bringing your body into a V shape, as available. As available, stretch or visualize this dynamic stretch through your hands and arms as well as your feet and legs as you lift and lengthen your torso and spine. Gaze forward or look down at your toes, keeping your head in line with your torso. Come out of the pose and return to Sitting Mountain.

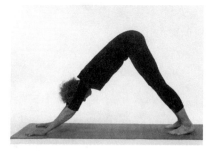

Downward-Facing Dog, on the mat

BENEFITS: PHYSICAL
- Stretches feet, calves, hamstrings, spine, shoulders, arms, and hands
- Strengthens spine, legs, and arms
- Builds core strength
- Improves digestion
- Increases blood and lymph circulation

BENEFITS: MENTAL
- Calms the mind
- Helps relieve stress and depression
- Builds confidence

EYE FOCUS
- Forward
- Ground

COUNTERPOSES
- Cobra Pose
- Backbends

Tips: As you come into the V-like shape, imagine that you are pushing the palms of your hands up toward the high seam and the soles of your feet onto a wall in front of you, lengthening and strengthening the limbs and muscles. To maintain balance, make sure you're not sitting too close to the front edge of the chair. If you need to make space for the belly, you can widen your legs into a V-shaped or L-shaped position. If you are lifting and raising your arms overhead, remember to soften and relax your shoulders to avoid strain. If you feel faint, lightheaded, or dizzy when raising your arms, keep your head level, looking forward with your eyes.

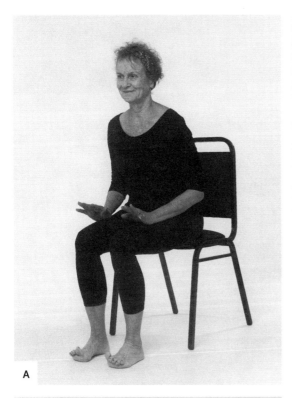

A

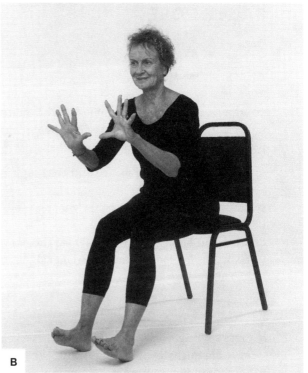

B

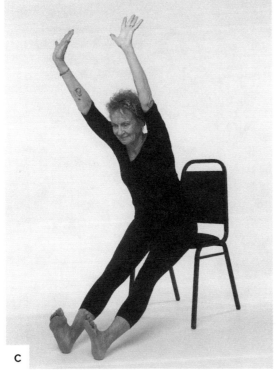

C

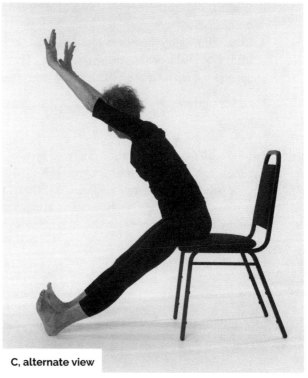

C, alternate view

EAGLE POSE

(Garudasana)

Begin in Sitting Mountain.

LOWER BODY: Move your right leg so that your right knee is in line with your navel and push down onto the three press points in your right foot. Choose to either:

A. Press your left leg and foot against your right leg, bringing the knees together;
B. Cross your left ankle over your right ankle, bringing the knees together; or
C. Cross your left leg over your right leg and, if available, hook your left foot behind your right calf, keeping your legs aligned.

UPPER BODY: Choose to either:

A. Cross your right wrist over the left and rest your hands on opposite thighs, palms facing down;
B. Raise your arms in front of your torso, palms facing inward, and cross your right wrist over the left at chest height; or
C. Cross your right elbow over your left elbow at the crease and, as available, either bring the backs of your forearms together, hook your thumbs, or bring your palms together.

Note: For option B, cross your arms and give yourself a hug if you wish!

Putting it all together: Once you find your level of flexibility, engage your leg muscles from your feet up into the core of your pelvis and squeeze your knees together. Lift and squeeze your arms and elbows together. Hinge forward (no more than forty-five degrees) and lengthen your spine. Gaze forward or down to the low seam. Return to Sitting Mountain and repeat on the other side.

Tip: Squeezing your legs and arms together gets the fluid between the joints moving, keeping them awake, active, and mobile. For the arms and hands, there are many options—feel free to experiment!

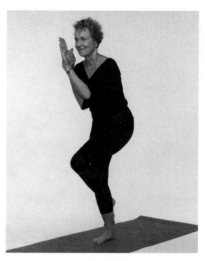

Eagle Pose, on the mat

BENEFITS: PHYSICAL
- Improves balance, coordination, and core strength
- Opens major joints of the body
- Strengthens feet, ankles, calves, and thighs
- Stretches wrists, arms, shoulders, chest, and back
- Improves circulation and digestion

BENEFITS: MENTAL
- Builds focus and concentration
- Fosters steadiness and grounding

EYE FOCUS
- Forward
- Low seam

COUNTERPOSE
- Sitting Mountain

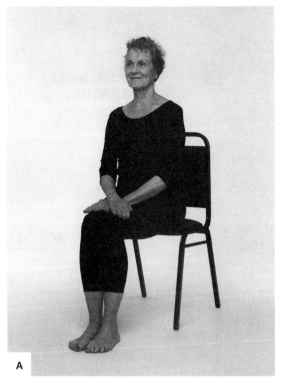

A

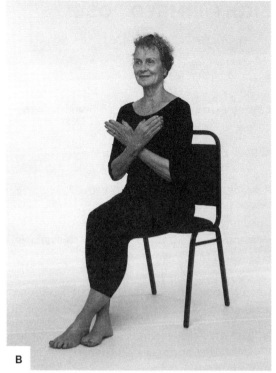

B

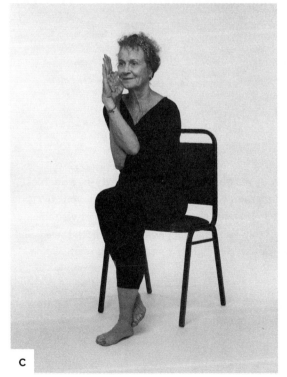

C

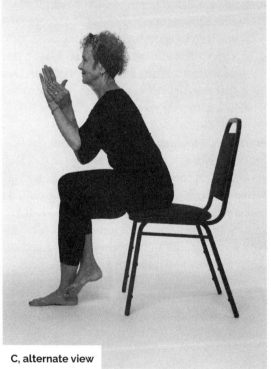

C, alternate view

EIGHT-LIMBED POSE

(Ashtanga Namaskara)

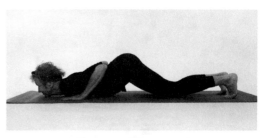

Eight-Limbed Pose, on the mat

Begin in Sitting Mountain.

LOWER BODY: With your legs hip-width apart, choose to either:

A. Keep the soles of your feet on the ground, pushing down onto the three press points;
B. Come onto the balls of your feet, pushing down onto the two press points; or
C. Remaining on the balls of your feet, move both feet back toward the chair up to six inches, as available, and push down onto the two press points.

UPPER BODY: Place the heels of your hands on your thighs and flex your hand up at the wrists. Choose to either:

A. Press the heels of your hands into your thighs as you engage and bring your elbows back and in close to your body;
B. Raise your flexed hands to chest height while engaging and bringing your elbows back and in close to your body as you lean forward slightly; or
C. Raise your flexed hands to shoulder height, draw your elbows down and in close to your body, and lean forward so that the backs of your hands press onto the front of or in line with your shoulders, as available.

> **BENEFITS: PHYSICAL**
> - Increases flexibility of the spine
> - Opens and strengthens chest, shoulders, and arms
> - Strengthens leg and core muscles
> - Stretches toes and feet
> - Improves balance
>
> **BENEFITS: MENTAL**
> - Increases focus and concentration
> - Lifts mood
>
> **EYE FOCUS**
> - Forward
> - High seam
>
> **COUNTERPOSES**
> - Sitting Mountain
> - Backbends

Putting it all together: Once you find your level of flexibility, press down onto the press points in your feet and engage your thigh and abdominal muscles. Hinge forward from your hips (no more than forty-five degrees), lifting the crown of your head toward the ceiling to lengthen your spine and the back of your neck as you relax your shoulders back and down. If available, jut your chin forward. Stretch or visualize stretching your fingers and press eight points of your body—chin, both palms, chest, both knees, and both feet—against an imaginary wall in front. Gaze forward or slightly up at the high seam. Come out of the pose and return to Sitting Mountain.

Tip: Sometimes instructed as knees-chest-chin on the mat, this transition pose in a Sun Salutation can energize both body and mind. It's often done in place of Cobra Pose.

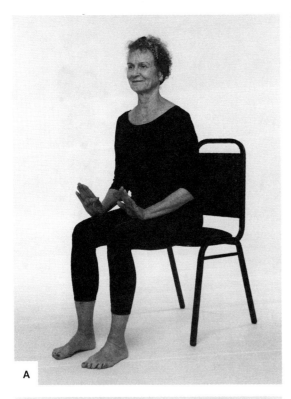

A

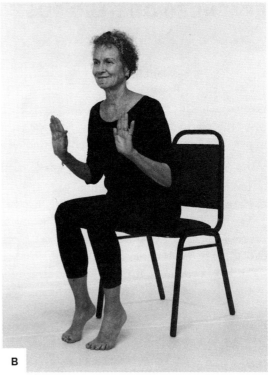

B

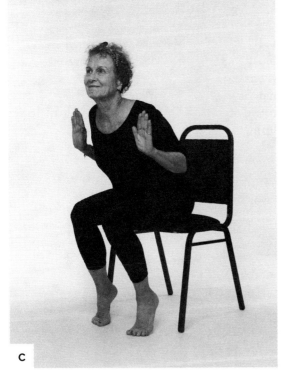

C

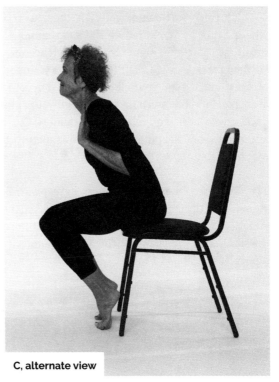

C, alternate view

EXTENDED ONE-LEG POSE

(Utthita Eka Padasana)

Begin in Sitting Mountain.

LOWER AND UPPER BODY: Since the hands are used to assist the legs in Extended One-Leg Pose, we set up the upper- and lower-body options together. Choose to either:

A. Come onto the ball of your left foot; place both hands under your left thigh, just behind your knee;

B. Place both hands under your left thigh, just behind your knee, and lift your leg off the ground, flexing your left foot and keeping your left knee bent; or

C. Place both hands under your left thigh, just behind your knee; flex your foot, lift your leg, and straighten it from the hip as available, no higher than ninety degrees.

Putting it all together: Once you find your level of flexibility, push down onto the three press points in your right foot and engage your right leg and foot muscles for balance. Come onto the ball of your left foot and place your hands under your left thigh, just behind your left knee. Keep your left leg where it is or lift it, extending and lengthening it from the hip as available—no higher than hip height—or visualize doing this. Flex your left foot, engage your abdominal muscles, and extend your elbows away from your body, as available. Lift your sternum to lengthen your spine and the back of your neck, and relax your shoulders. Gaze forward or at the low seam, keeping your neck long. Return to Sitting Mountain and repeat on the other side.

Tips: Extended One-Leg Pose offers a great warm-up. It also strengthens the core muscles and increases balance. In any variation, you may want to try extending your arms out to the sides, with your palms facing up and hands in Jnana Mudra, if available.

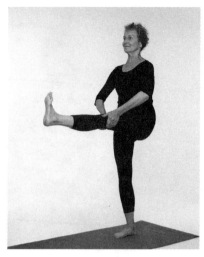

Extended One-Leg Pose, on the mat

BENEFITS: PHYSICAL
- Increases balance and core awareness
- Strengthens abdominal, leg, arm, and foot muscles
- Lengthens spine
- Tones and strengthens hands, arms, and shoulders
- Increases postural awareness
- Stretches hamstrings and calves
- Supports knee health
- Enhances circulation and digestion

BENEFITS: MENTAL
- Improves focus
- Cultivates confidence

EYE FOCUS
- Forward
- Low seam

COUNTERPOSE
- Sitting Mountain

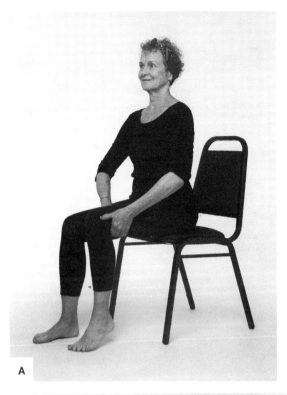

A

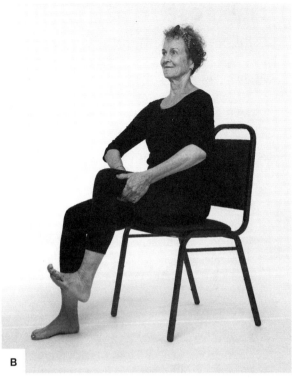

B

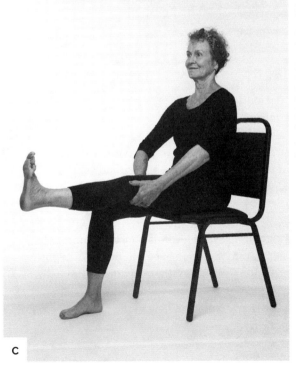

C

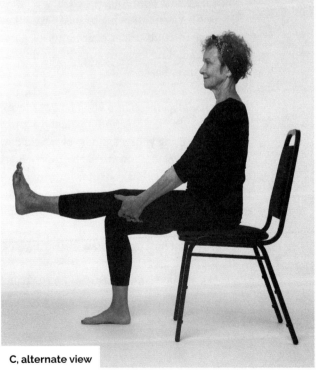

C, alternate view

FISH POSE

(Matsyasana)

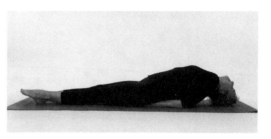

Fish Pose, on the mat

Begin in Sitting Mountain.

LOWER BODY: With your legs hip-width apart, choose to either:

A. Keep the soles of your feet on the ground, pushing down onto the three press points;
B. Bring your legs together, in line with your navel, and slide your feet forward, with the soles pushing down onto the ground; or
C. With your legs together, slide your feet as far forward as available, with the soles pushing down onto the ground, and point your toes.

UPPER BODY: Choose to either:

A. Place your hands on your waist or hips and slightly draw your elbows back and toward each other;
B. Place your palms down on the chair seat next to your buttocks, with your fingers pointing forward and your elbows back and drawing toward each other; or
C. Bring your hands under your buttocks, palms down, with fingers pointing forward and elbows drawn back and closer toward each other.

Putting it all together: Once you find your level of flexibility, engage your leg muscles from the feet up into the core of your pelvis. Bring your shoulders back and down and draw your shoulder blades toward each other. Lengthen your tailbone and extend your pelvis forward toward your knees. Lift your sternum, engage your upper-body muscles, and extend your jaw forward. Gaze forward or lift your chin slightly to look at the high seam (not the ceiling). Come out of the pose and return to Sitting Mountain.

Tips: Instead of jutting your jaw forward, you can extend just your lower jaw forward and smile. With options B and C, another variation for your hands is to flip them over and press down onto the backs of your hands instead of on the palms, stretching and strengthening different muscles of your hands and arms.

Avoid dropping your head too far back to protect the arterial blood flow in the neck.

BENEFITS: PHYSICAL
- Strengthens muscles of shoulders, upper back, neck, and jaw
- Opens hips, abdomen, chest, and throat
- Strengthens legs and feet
- Stimulates digestion and circulation

BENEFITS: MENTAL
- Relieves stress and fatigue
- Lifts mood

EYE FOCUS
- Forward
- High seam

COUNTERPOSES
- Forward Fold
- Spinal Twist

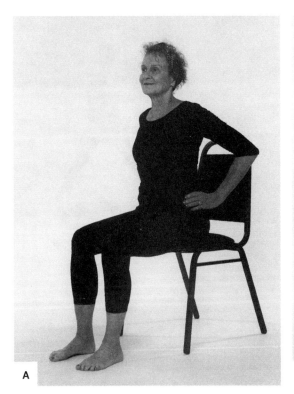

A

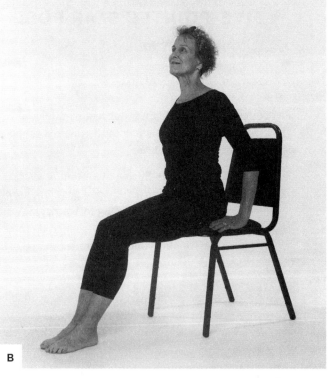

B

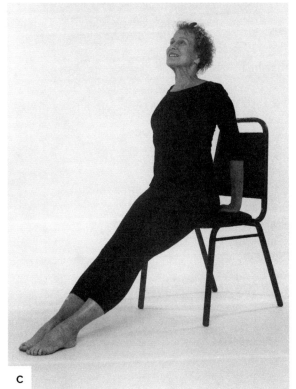

C

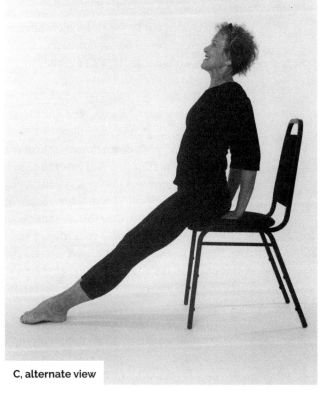

C, alternate view

FIVE-POINTED STAR POSE

(Utthita Tadasana)

Start in Sitting Mountain.

LOWER BODY: Keeping your feet parallel and your toes facing forward, push down onto the three press points in your feet and choose to either:

A. Leave your legs in Sitting Mountain;
B. Bring your legs into a V-shaped position, keeping your feet parallel and your toes facing forward; or
C. Bring your legs into a wider V-shaped or an L-shaped position, keeping your feet parallel and your toes facing forward.

UPPER BODY: Straighten your arms, as available, down by your sides, in line with your torso. Rotate your palms and inner arms to face your body and, from there, choose to either:

A. Lift your arms out to the side, slightly away from your body, palms facing inward;
B. Lift your arms out to the side a bit higher so they're at waist height, palms facing down; or
C. Lift your arms out to the side at shoulder height, palms facing down.

Putting it all together: Once you find your level of flexibility, engage your thigh and abdominal muscles. Point your toes forward and push down onto the three press points in your feet. Lift the crown of your head toward the ceiling to lengthen your spine and the back of your neck as you relax your shoulders back and down. Lift your sternum and, as available, stretch or visualize this dynamic stretch through your hands and arms; spread your fingers and imagine your nose, palms, and toes (or your head, arms, and legs) as five points of a star. Gaze forward or up at the high seam. Come out of the pose and return to Sitting Mountain.

Tips: Included as a transition pose in a Moon Salutation, this variation of Mountain Pose can bolster strength in both body and mind.

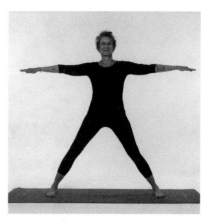

Five-Pointed Star Pose, on the mat

BENEFITS: PHYSICAL
- Aligns spine and improves posture
- Opens and strengthens chest, shoulders, and arm muscles
- Strengthens muscles of feet, legs, and abdomen
- Stimulates circulation
- Improves balance

BENEFITS: MENTAL
- Increases focus and concentration
- Lifts mood and relieves stress

EYE FOCUS
- Forward
- High seam

COUNTERPOSE
- Sitting Mountain

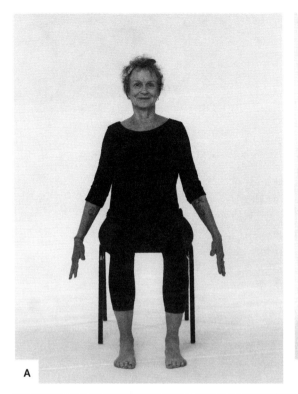

A

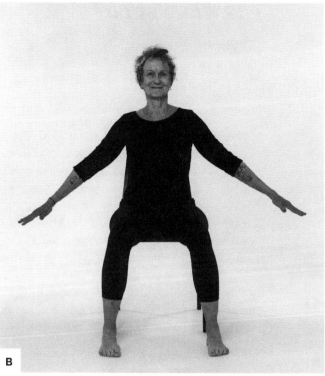

B

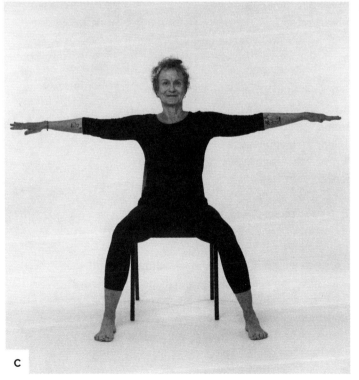

C

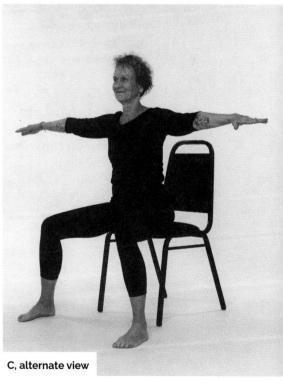

C, alternate view

FORWARD FOLD

(Pashchimottanasana)

Begin in Sitting Mountain.

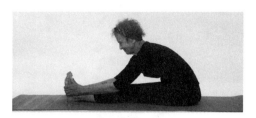

Forward Fold, on the mat

LOWER BODY: Choose to either:

A. Keep your legs in Sitting Mountain and lift your toes, coming up onto your heels, as available;
B. Extend your legs forward, keeping your knees bent and coming up onto your heels with feet flexed at the ankles; or
C. Extend your legs forward and straighten your knees as far as available, remaining on your heels with your feet flexed at the ankles.

UPPER BODY: Place your hands on your thighs, palms down, and hinge forward at the hips as available, keeping your back lengthened. Choose to either:

A. Slide your hands down the front or along the outside of your legs, stopping near your knees;
B. Slide your hands down your legs, stopping at the middle of your calves (or anywhere on your legs); or
C. Slide your hands all the way down your legs toward your feet, holding on to either your ankles, heels, or toes.

Putting it all together: Once you find your level of flexibility, engage the muscles of your legs and buttocks. Flex your feet and push your heels down onto the ground. As you hinge forward, lift the crown of your head to lengthen your spine. Place your hands with your palms down on your thighs, knees, calves, ankles, or toes—anywhere on your legs or feet—or visualize this. Gaze forward, at the low seam, or on the ground, maintaining the length in your torso. Come out of the pose and return to Sitting Mountain.

BENEFITS: PHYSICAL
- Stretches back body—hamstrings, calves, and lower back
- Increases length and flexibility in spine
- Stimulates internal organs and digestion
- Increases blood and lymph circulation
- Strengthens thighs and knees
- Improves balance
- May alleviate menopause symptoms, insomnia, and headache

BENEFITS: MENTAL
- Calms the mind
- Relieves stress and depression
- Reduces fatigue and anxiety

EYE FOCUS
- Forward
- Low seam
- Ground

COUNTERPOSES
- Sitting Mountain
- Backbends

Tips: If you have any bone loss, keep your torso lengthened to avoid rounding your spine. If you need to make space for the belly, you can widen your legs into a V-shaped or L-shaped position. If you feel faint, lightheaded, or dizzy and this pose does not feel comfortable, keep your head above your heart, moving into whatever level of flexibility feels doable and visualizing the rest. For a more restorative, relaxing option, lower your head and close your eyes, placing pillows or a bolster on your lap, if that feels good. Explore other forward-fold poses, such as Child's Pose (page 92), using our levels of flexibility.

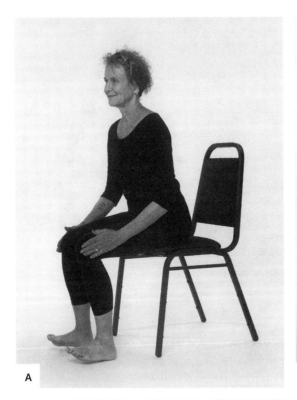

A

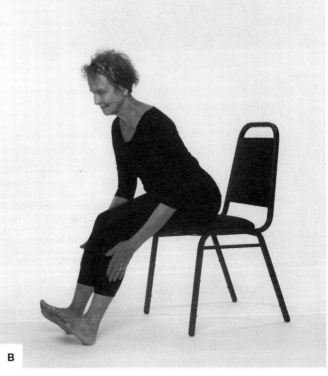

B

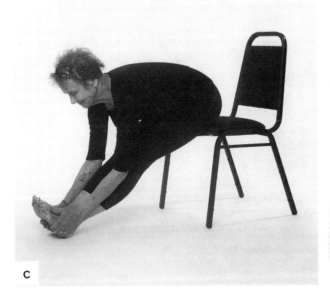

C

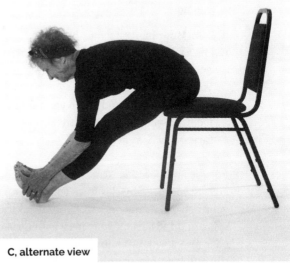

C, alternate view

GATE POSE

(Parighasana)

Begin in Sitting Mountain.

LOWER BODY: Choose to either:

A. Leave your left leg in Sitting Mountain and move your right leg into a V-shaped position, keeping your right knee aligned over your right ankle and pushing down onto the three press points;

B. Come onto the ball of your left foot and move your right leg into an L-shaped position, keeping your right knee aligned over your right ankle; push down onto the two press points in your left foot and the three press points in your right foot; or

C. Remaining on the ball of your left foot, move your left foot back toward the chair up to six inches, pushing down onto the two press points; extend your right leg straight out to the right as available, keeping your right foot flat on the ground, toes and knee pointing forward, pushing down onto the three press points.

UPPER BODY: Lean your torso to the right and choose to either:

A. Bring your hands to your hips;

B. Place your right hand on your right thigh, palm facing down; bend your left elbow and place your left hand on your left shoulder; or

C. Slide your right hand down your extended right leg and lengthen your left arm to arch up and overhead, palm facing down, as available.

Putting it all together: Once you find your level of flexibility, engage your leg muscles from your feet up into the core of your pelvis. Lift the crown of your head to lengthen your spine and the back of your neck as you relax your shoulders back and down. Lift your sternum and begin to extend, tilt, and lengthen your torso to the right, pushing your feet down onto the ground and drawing your left shoulder back.

(CONTINUED ON NEXT SPREAD)

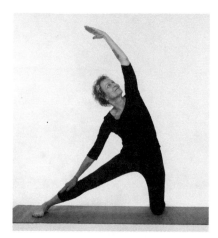

Gate Pose, on the mat

BENEFITS: PHYSICAL
- Lengthens spine and side body
- Stretches muscles in feet, legs, groin, ribcage, arms, and neck
- Opens throat, chest, shoulders, and hips
- Strengthens and tones legs and core muscles
- Improves respiration

BENEFITS: MENTAL
- Builds focus and attention
- Relieves stress

EYE FOCUS
- High seam
- Forward
- Downward

COUNTERPOSES
- Sitting Mountain
- Forward Fold

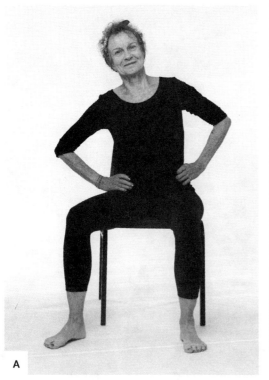

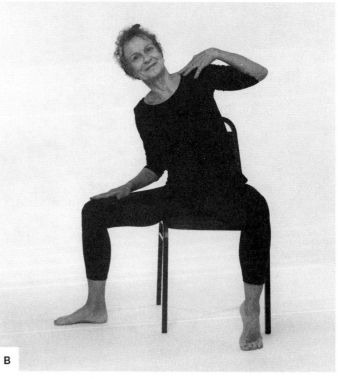

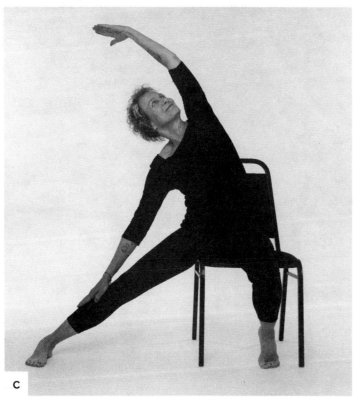

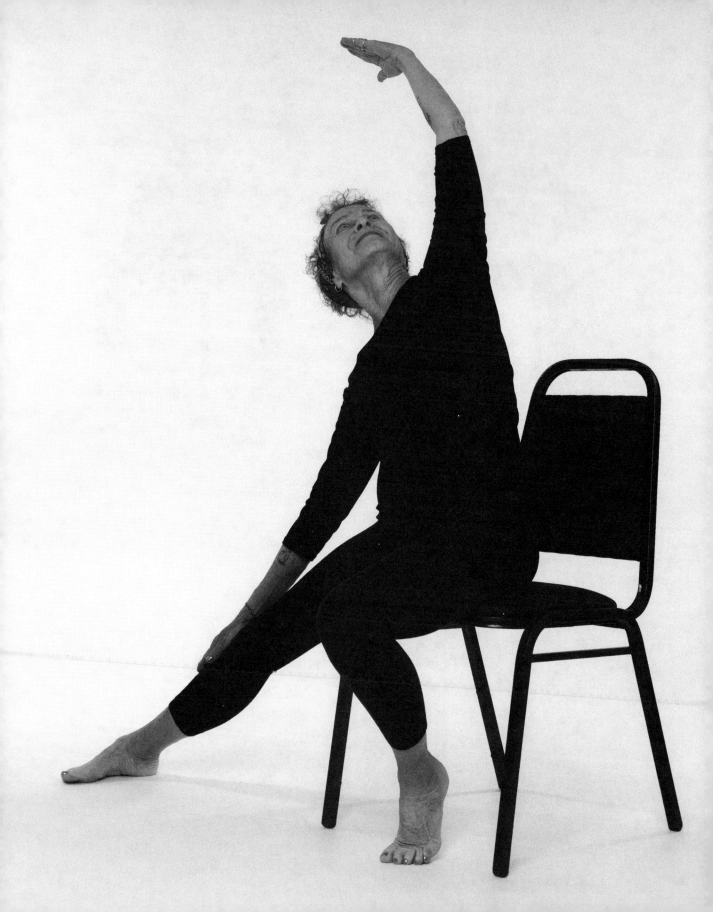

Stretch through your left arm and hand overhead and your right arm and hand down on the right side, as available. Gaze up to the high seam, forward, or down onto the ground. Return to Sitting Mountain and repeat on the other side.

Tips: Also known as Beam Pose, this posture offers the chance to stretch most muscles of the body.

Remember to mix and match the sides of the body as well as upper- and lower-body options. For example, you might want to keep one hand on your hip while lengthening your other arm up and over, if this feels comfortable; move into whatever level of flexibility feels doable and visualize the rest. If you are lifting and raising an arm overhead, remember to soften and relax your shoulder to avoid strain. If you feel faint, lightheaded, or dizzy when raising an arm, keep your head level, looking forward with your eyes and not up.

Gate Pose (option C, alternative view)

HALF FORWARD FOLD

(Ardha Uttanasana)

Begin in Sitting Mountain.

LOWER BODY: Keep your legs in Sitting Mountain, pushing down onto the three press points in your feet.

UPPER BODY: Keeping your arms shoulder-width apart, place your hands on the outside of your thighs, palms facing inward. Hinging forward, choose to either:

A. Bend your elbows and bring your hands along the outsides of your legs toward your knees;
B. With elbows bent, bring your hands down the outside of your legs until they reach midcalf; or
C. With elbows bent, bring your hands down the outside of your legs until they reach your ankles.

Putting it all together: Once you find your level of flexibility, engage the muscles of your legs and buttocks and, as you begin to hinge forward at your hips, lift your sternum to lengthen your spine and the back of your neck, and draw your shoulders back and down. Bring your hands down outside or onto your thighs, knees, calves, or ankles—anywhere on your legs or feet—or visualize this. Gaze forward or down at the low seam or onto the ground, maintaining the length in the front of your torso as well as your spine. Come out of the pose and return to Sitting Mountain.

Tips: Also known as Halfway Lift, this pose follows Upward Salute in a Sun Salutation. It can also be practiced with your arms straightened and your hands touching the front of your legs, feet, or ground, as available. If you have any bone loss, keep your torso lengthened to avoid rounding your spine. If you need to make space for your belly, you can widen your legs into a V-shaped or L-shaped position. If you feel faint, lightheaded, or dizzy and this pose does not feel comfortable, keep your head above your heart, moving into whatever level of flexibility feels doable and visualizing the rest.

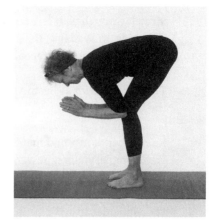

Half Forward Fold, on the mat

BENEFITS: PHYSICAL
- Increases spinal strength and flexibility
- Stretches front body
- Improves circulation and digestion
- Strengthens balance

BENEFITS: MENTAL
- Calms the mind
- Relieves stress and depression

EYE FOCUS
- Forward
- Low seam
- Downward

COUNTERPOSES
- Sitting Mountain
- Backbends

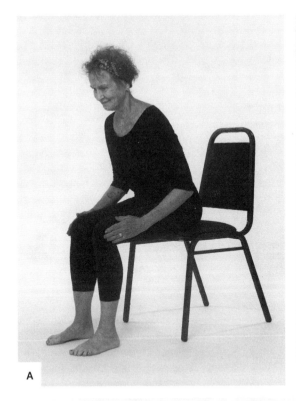

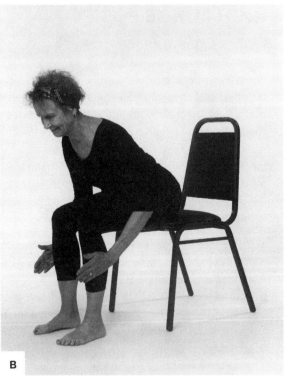

A

B

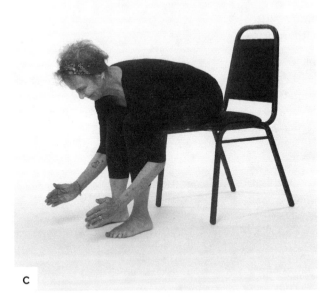

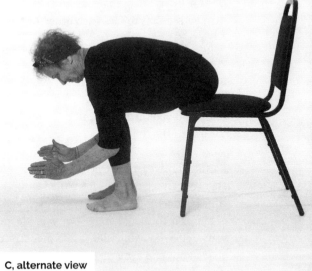

C

C, alternate view

HIGH LUNGE POSE

(Ashta Chandrasana)

Begin in Sitting Mountain. Turn and face the right side of the chair and reestablish Sitting Mountain. Keep your right buttock on the chair; your left buttock may extend off the chair as needed, keeping both sit bones on the chair.

LOWER BODY: With your right leg in Sitting Mountain, push down onto the three press points in your right foot. Coming onto the ball of your left foot and pushing down onto the two press points, choose to either:

A. Bring your left foot beside the outside of the front right chair leg, keeping your knee bent and adjusting your buttocks on the chair as needed;

B. Extend your left leg back farther and lower your left knee down from your hip toward the ground, adjusting your buttocks on the chair as needed; or

C. Lengthen your left leg back even farther, either keeping your knee bent or straightening it, adjusting your buttocks on the chair as needed.

UPPER BODY: Keeping your arms shoulder-width apart, turn your palms to face each other. Choose to either:

A. Rest the outside of your hands on your thighs, elbows bent and in close to your body;

B. Keeping your elbows bent, lift your hands to chest or head height; or

C. Extend your arms straight out from your shoulders and up toward the ceiling.

Putting it all together: Once you find your level of flexibility, engage your leg muscles from the feet up into the core of your pelvis. Draw your shoulders back and down, lengthening your torso and spine. Lift your sternum and engage your upper-body muscles, and either stretch or visualize your hands and arms stretching long, keeping your body vertical. Gaze forward or up to the high seam. To come out of the pose, return to Sitting Mountain on the right side of the chair before moving to the front of the chair into Sitting Mountain. Repeat on the other side.

(CONTINUED ON NEXT SPREAD)

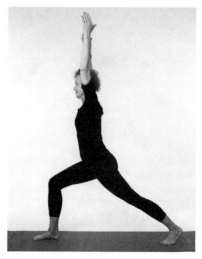

High Lunge Pose, on the mat

BENEFITS: PHYSICAL
- Strengthens arches, ankles, knees, legs, back, and arms
- Stretches hips, chest, shoulders, and arms
- Supports knee strength and stability
- Increases pelvic floor and core muscle strength
- Stimulates digestion and circulation
- Relieves sciatica and back pain
- Improves balance

BENEFITS: MENTAL
- Builds concentration and focus
- Develops attention and motivation
- Energizes mood

EYE FOCUS
- Forward
- High seam

COUNTERPOSES
- Sitting Mountain
- Downward-Facing Dog

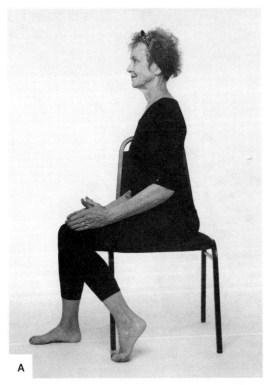

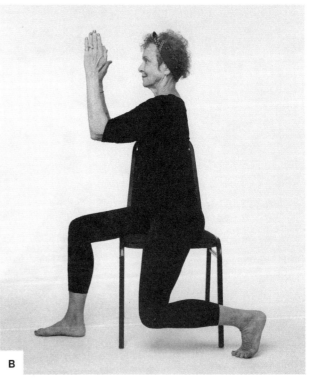

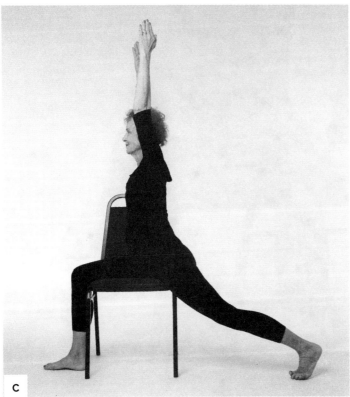

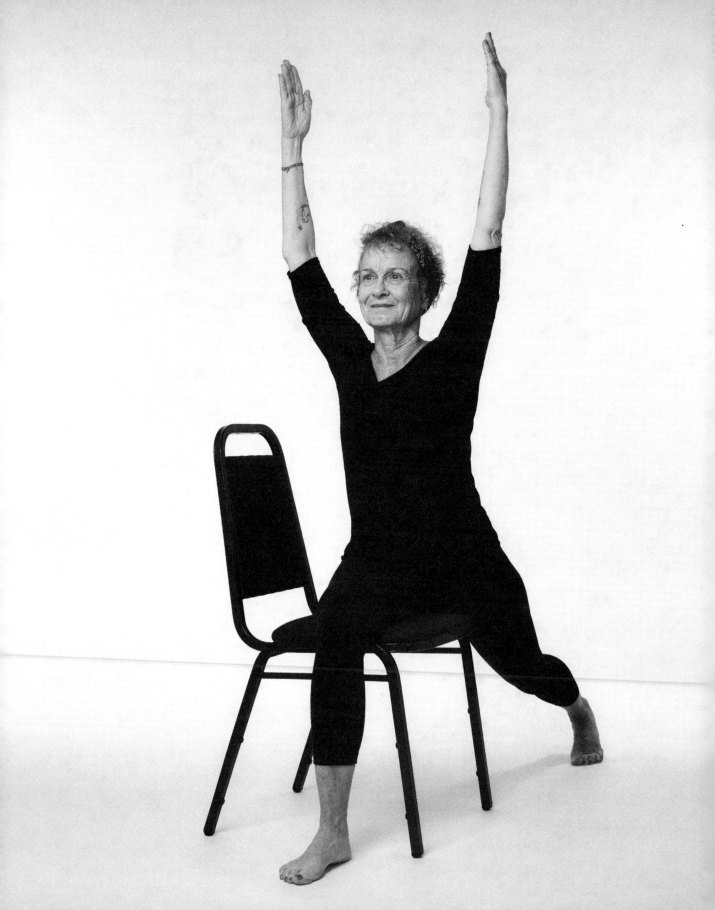

Tips: Yoga offers many variations of lunge poses. If you prefer to face forward on the chair or are using a chair with arms, see Lunge Pose (page 140). For increased back strengthening, add back-bending movements by following the lower-body instructions above and the upper-body instructions for King Pigeon Pose (Eka Pada Rajakapotasana) (page 132), with hands together or shoulder-width apart; these variations are known as Low Lunge Pose and Crescent Lunge Pose (Anjaneyasana). If you are lifting and raising your arms overhead, remember to soften and relax your shoulders to avoid strain. If you feel faint, lightheaded, or dizzy when raising your arms, keep your head level, looking forward with your eyes, not up.

High Lunge Pose (option C, alternative view)

HUMBLE WARRIOR

(Baddha Virabhadrasana)

Begin in Sitting Mountain. Turn and face the right side of the chair and reestablish Sitting Mountain. Keep your right buttock on the chair; your left buttock may extend off the chair as needed, keeping both sit bones on the chair.

LOWER BODY: With your right leg in Sitting Mountain, press down onto the three press points in your right foot. Choose to either:

A. Bring your left leg into a V-shaped position;

B. Bring your left leg into an L-shaped position; or

C. Bring your left leg into an extended position, as available. Turn your left foot to face forward with the sole flat on the ground, adjusting your buttocks on the chair as needed.

UPPER BODY: Choose to either:

A. Bring your right hand to hold on to the back of the chair seat and your left hand to hold on to the front of the chair seat; hinge slightly forward from your hips over your right leg;

B. Clasp your hands behind your back and hinge farther forward over your right leg from your hips; or

C. Clasp your hands behind your back and hinge farther forward from your hips, bringing your chest toward your right thigh and raising your arms up and over as far as available.

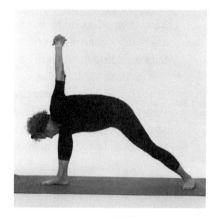

Humble Warrior, on the mat

BENEFITS: PHYSICAL
- Opens back, groin, hips, shoulders, and neck
- Stretches chest, arms, and hands
- Strengthens feet, knees, and legs
- Improves balance

BENEFITS: MENTAL
- Builds focus and confidence
- Can lift and calm mood

EYE FOCUS
- Downward

COUNTERPOSES
- Reverse Warrior
- Warrior II

Putting it all together: Once you find your level of flexibility, engage your leg muscles from the feet up into the core of your pelvis. Draw your shoulders back and down, lengthening your torso and spine. Gently twist to the right so that your torso is facing your right leg. Now lift your sternum and engage your upper-body muscles, stretching your arms and hands as available. Hinging from your hips, fold over your right leg to your level of flexibility. Gaze down as your neck allows. To come out of the pose, return to Sitting Mountain on the right side of the chair before moving to the front of the chair into Sitting Mountain. Repeat on the other side.

(CONTINUED ON NEXT SPREAD)

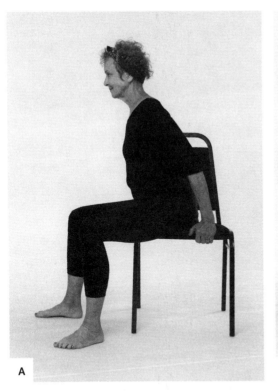

A

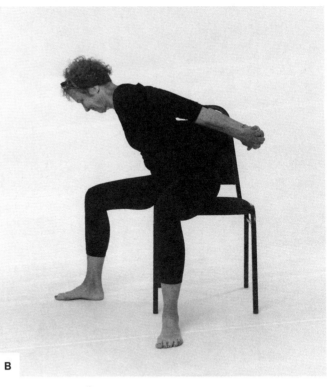

B

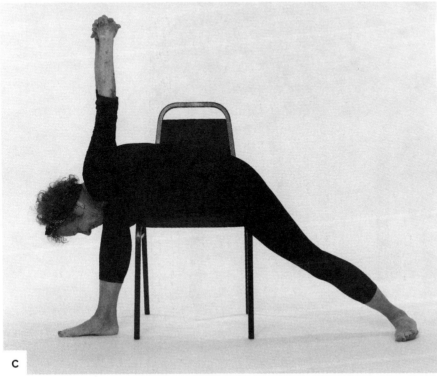

C

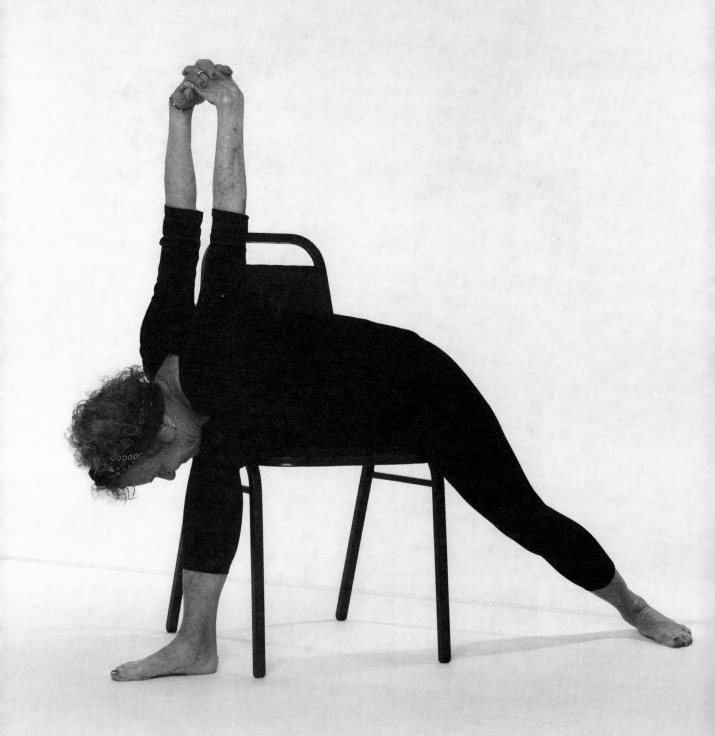

Tips: With its combination of lower-body engagement and forward folding of the upper body, this pose can both energize and calm the body and mind. Also known as Bound or Devotional Warrior, Humble Warrior can be done facing forward on the chair as an alternative, following the lower-body instructions for Warrior II (page 178). On a chair with arms, follow the lower-body options in Squat Pose (Malasana) (page 158)—Sitting Mountain legs, V-shaped leg, and L-shaped leg; for the upper body, option A for Humble Warrior works best. If you need to make space for your belly, you can hinge forward into the opening between the legs instead of over the front leg. When lifting and raising your arms back and overhead, remember to soften and relax your shoulders to avoid strain. If you feel faint, lightheaded, or dizzy, remain upright and keep your head level, looking forward with your eyes; move into whatever level of flexibility feels doable and visualize the rest.

Humble Warrior (option C, alternative view)

KING PIGEON POSE

(Eka Pada Rajakapotasana)

Begin in Sitting Mountain. Turn and face the right side of the chair and reestablish Sitting Mountain. Keep your right buttock on the chair; your left buttock may extend off the chair as needed, keeping both sit bones on the chair.

LOWER BODY: With your right leg in Sitting Mountain, push down onto the three press points in your right foot and choose to either:

A. Come onto the ball of your left foot, positioning your left foot beside the outside of the front right chair leg, keeping your knee bent and the sole of your right foot flat on the ground;

B. Extend your left leg back farther, lowering your left knee down from your hip toward the ground and coming onto the top of your left foot by curling your toes under and resting the front or top of the toes on the ground; turn your right foot onto its outside edge, little-toe side down; or

C. Lengthen your left leg back as available, keeping your knee bent or straightened while remaining on top of your foot; turn your right foot onto its outside edge, little-toe side down.

Note: An alternative for the extended leg in options B and C is to come onto the ball of your foot instead of the top and push down onto the two press points.

UPPER BODY: Bringing the palms of your hands together, choose to either:

A. Place the knuckles of your thumbs onto your sternum or slightly away from your body;

B. Lift your arms until your hands are in line with your face or the top of your head, keeping the elbows bent; hinge back slightly from your hips; or

C. Lift your arms, straightening them up next to your ears and reaching up, as available; hinge farther back from the hips.

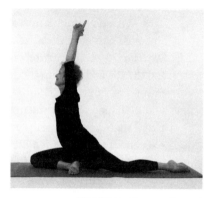

King Pigeon Pose, on the mat

BENEFITS: PHYSICAL
- Opens thighs, hips, psoas, chest, and shoulders
- Stretches feet, thighs, and back
- Tones abdomen and arms
- Stimulates digestion and circulation
- Improves balance

BENEFITS: MENTAL
- Develops focus
- Reduces stress
- Cultivates energy

EYE FOCUS
- Forward
- High seam

COUNTERPOSE
- Forward Fold

(CONTINUED ON NEXT SPREAD)

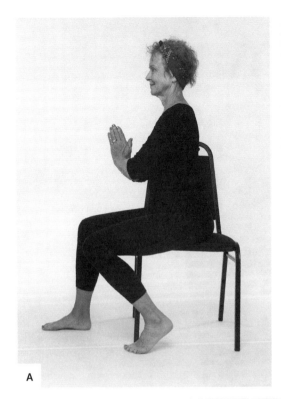

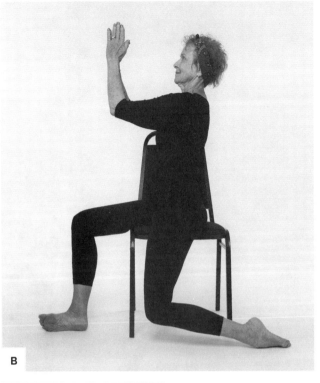

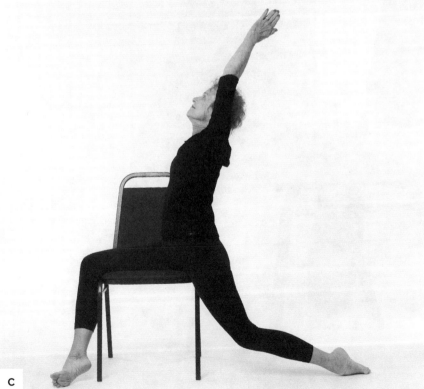

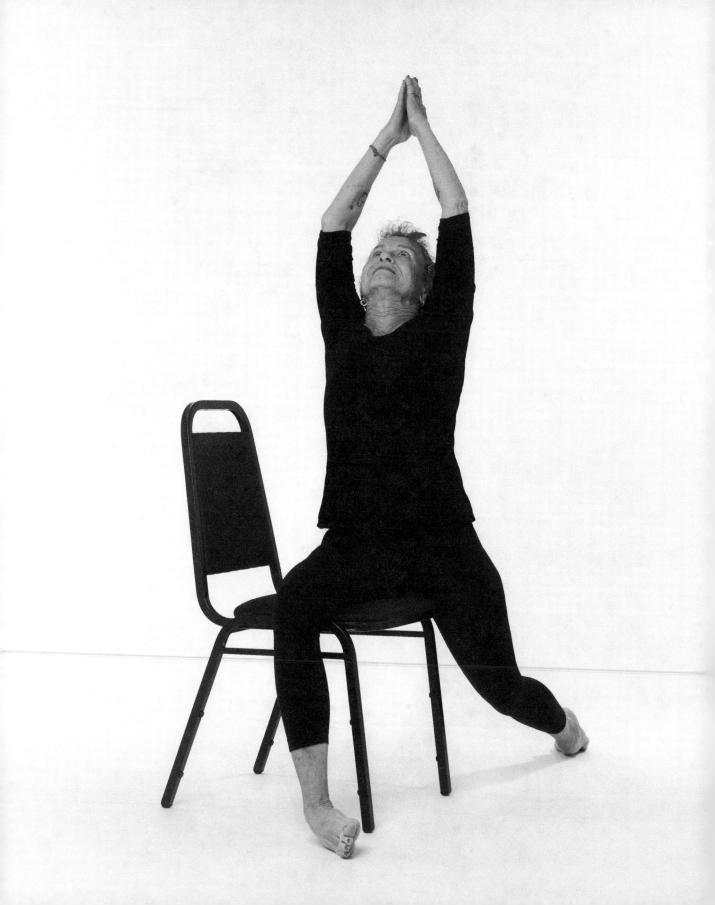

Putting it all together: Once you find your level of flexibility, engage your leg muscles from your feet up into the core of your pelvis. Engaging your abdominal and upper-body muscles, stretch your hands, arms, and front body as you hinge your torso back from your hips as available. Gaze forward or up to the high seam. To come out of the pose, return to Sitting Mountain on the right side of the chair before moving to the front of the chair into Sitting Mountain. Repeat on the other side.

Tips: Also known as One-Legged King Pigeon Pose, this posture on a chair allows you to focus on its back-bending qualities—strengthening the back, lengthening the front of the body, and releasing the hips as well as energizing both the body and the mind. When moving to the side of the chair, use your hands to hold the seat of the chair for safety and stability. See Pigeon Pose (Kapotasana) (page 144) for a calming variation of this posture. When lifting and raising your arms overhead, remember to soften and relax your shoulders to avoid strain. If you feel faint, lightheaded, or dizzy when raising your arms, keep your head level, looking forward with your eyes, not up; move into whatever level of flexibility feels doable and visualize the rest.

King Pigeon Pose (option C, alternative view)

KNEE-TO-CHEST POSE

(Eka Pada Apanasana)

Begin in Sitting Mountain.

LOWER AND UPPER BODY: Since the hands are used to assist the legs in Knee-to-Chest Pose, we set up the upper- and lower-body options together. Choose to either:

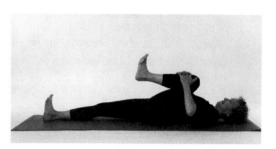

Knee-to-Chest Pose, on the mat

A. Keep your right leg in Sitting Mountain and come onto the ball of your left foot; as you hinge forward, bring your left hand just below your left knee and place your right hand on your right thigh, palm down; sit up tall with the ball of your left foot or the toes on the ground and gently pull your left knee toward your torso;

B. Extend your right leg slightly in front of you and come onto your right heel; as you hinge forward, clasp your left leg just below your left knee with both hands and lift it off the ground; sit up tall and pull your left knee toward your torso, flexing both feet; or

C. Lengthen your right leg forward as far as available and flex your right foot; with your hands clasped under your left knee, pull it as high as available toward your left armpit, flexing your left foot.

Putting it all together: Once you find your level of flexibility, extend your right leg forward, straightening it as long as available. Press the heel of your right foot onto the ground and engage your leg and foot muscles for balance. Lift your sternum to lengthen your spine and the back of your neck, and relax your shoulders back and down. As you move your left knee toward your chest, engage your abdominal muscles, press through your right leg, and sit up as tall as available. Extend your elbows away from your body or pull them in close. Gaze forward or at the low seam, keeping the neck long. Return to Sitting Mountain and repeat on the other side.

Tip: When you do this posture, aptly known as Wind-Relieving Pose (Pavanamuktasana), start on your right side in line with intestinal flow to support digestion.

BENEFITS: PHYSICAL
- Stretches knees, lower back, hips, legs, and arms
- Eases digestion and lower back pain
- Stimulates lymphatic flow

BENEFITS: MENTAL
- Reduces stress

EYE FOCUS
- Forward
- Low seam

COUNTERPOSES
- Sitting Mountain
- Yoga Rest Pose

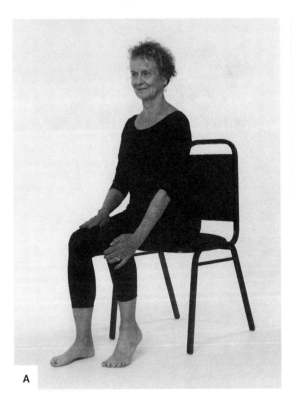

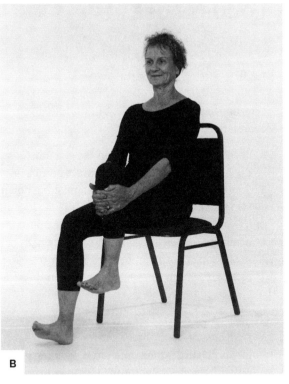

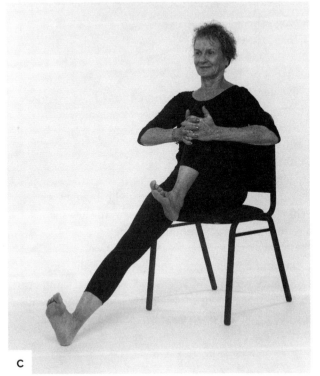

A

B

C

C, alternate view

LOCUST POSE

(Shalabhasana)

Begin in Sitting Mountain

LOWER BODY: With your legs hip-width apart, choose to either:

A. Keep the soles of your feet on the ground, pushing down onto the three press points;
B. Come onto the balls of your feet, pushing down onto the two press points; or
C. Move both feet back toward the chair up to six inches, as available, and either come up onto the balls of your feet or the top of both feet by curling your toes under and resting the front or top of your toes on the ground.

UPPER BODY: Choose to either:

A. Take hold of the front legs of your chair (or the front edges of your chair seat) on both sides, keeping your elbows either bent or straightened; hinge slightly forward from your hips;
B. Take hold of the chair seat on both sides, keeping your elbows either bent or straightened; hinge farther forward from your hips; or
C. Take hold of the back of the chair and hinge farther forward from your hips (no more than forty-five degrees); stretch and straighten your arms as available.

Putting it all together: Once you find your level of flexibility, engage your leg and abdominal muscles from your feet up into the core of your pelvis. Lift your sternum to lengthen your spine and the back of your neck, drawing your shoulders back and down and bringing your shoulder blades toward each other. Raise your chin slightly. Gaze forward, down to the low seam, or up to the high seam. Come out of the pose and return to Sitting Mountain.

Tips: Holding on to the sides of the chair and using your body weight to hinge forward allows you to maintain or build bone mass in the upper body. Balance permitting, release your arms back and out like a bird or airplane and fly! If you have any bone loss, keep your torso lengthened to avoid rounding your spine. If you need to make space for the belly, you can open your legs wider into a V-shaped or L-shaped position.

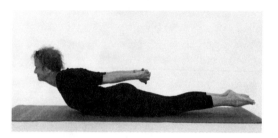

Locust Pose, on the mat

BENEFITS: PHYSICAL
- Strengthens legs, shoulders, arms, and hands
- Lengthens spine and back
- Opens chest, shoulders, and throat
- Increases circulation and respiration
- Improves bone mass and posture

BENEFITS: MENTAL
- Relieves stress and fatigue
- Lifts mood

EYE FOCUS
- Forward
- Low seam
- High seam

COUNTERPOSES
- Sitting Mountain
- Child's Pose

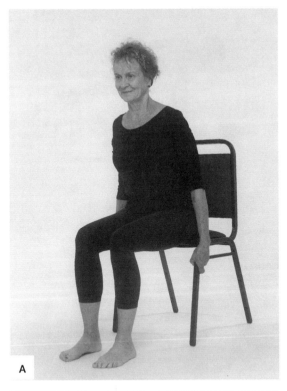

A

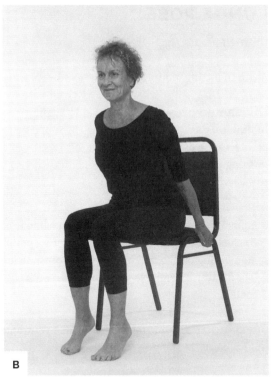

B

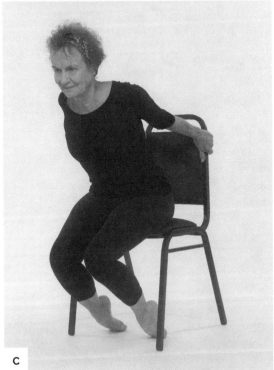

C

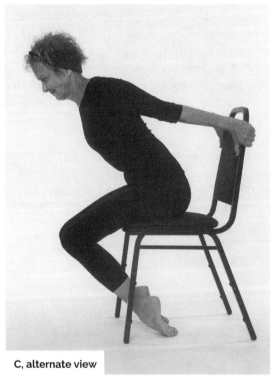

C, alternate view

LUNGE POSE

(Banarasana)

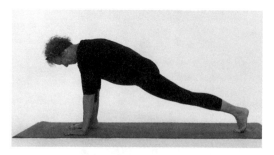

Lunge Pose, on the mat

Begin in Sitting Mountain.

LOWER BODY: Keep your right leg in Sitting Mountain, pushing down onto the three press points. Come onto the ball of your left foot, pushing down onto the two press points. Choose to either:

A. Stay in that position;
B. Remaining on the ball of the left foot, slide it back a few inches, pushing down onto the two press points; or
C. Remaining on the ball of your left foot, slide it back up to six inches, as available, pushing down onto the two press points.

UPPER BODY: In all three options, place your hands on your thighs, palms facing down.

Putting it all together: Once you find your level of flexibility, engage the muscles of your thighs and buttocks by pushing down onto the press points in your feet. Lift your sternum and hinge forward from your hips as far as available (no more than forty-five degrees). Draw your shoulders back and down, expand your chest, and keep your spine lengthened. Gaze forward or down at the low seam or the ground. Return to Sitting Mountain and repeat on the other side.

Tips: Sometimes called Runner's Lunge, this posture often appears in Sun Salutations as a transition between Forward Fold (pages 116) and Plank Pose (pages 146). For related poses, see High Lunge Pose (pages 124) and Revolved Lunge Pose (pages 154).

BENEFITS: PHYSICAL
- Strengthens and tones feet, ankles, and leg muscles
- Supports knee strength and stability
- Increases pelvic floor and core muscle strength
- Expands chest
- Can relieve sciatica and back pain
- Improves balance

BENEFITS: MENTAL
- Relaxes the mind
- Lifts and calms mood

EYE FOCUS
- Forward
- Low seam
- Downward

COUNTERPOSE
- Sitting Mountain

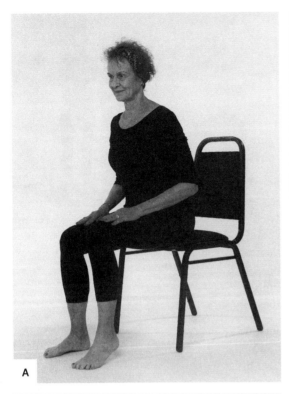

A

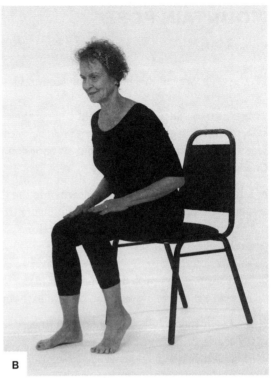

B

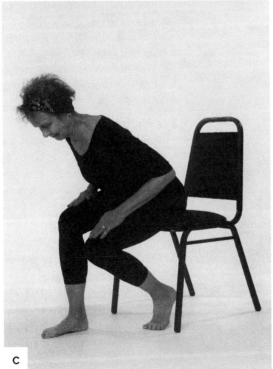

C

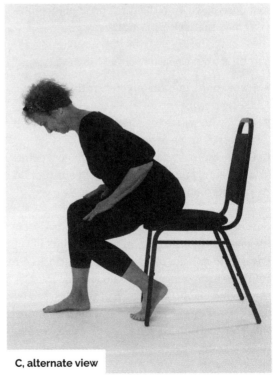

C, alternate view

MOUNTAIN POSE

(Tadasana)

On the chair, we call this pose Sitting Mountain.

LOWER BODY: Sit as near the front edge of the chair as feels safe, with your legs hip-width apart and the soles of your feet flat on the ground. Anchor your sit bones on the chair. Choose to either:

A. Lift your toes and lightly push down onto the three press points in the soles of your feet, then release your toes;

B. Lift your toes and push down onto the three press points in the soles of your feet with moderate pressure, then release your toes; or

C. Lift your toes and push down firmly onto the three press points in the soles of your feet, then release your toes.

Note: If your thighs fully touch and your knees face outward in a V shape, bring your heels in line with each other and your knees over your ankles as available. Allow your feet to point out in the same direction as your knees, lift your toes, and push down onto the three press points in the soles of your feet, then release your toes.

UPPER BODY: Choose to either:

A. Place your hands on top of your thighs, your palms facing down;

B. Bring your palms together in front of your rib cage, fingers pointing forward; or

C. Bring your palms together, your fingers pointing up, and gently press the knuckles of your thumbs onto your sternum.

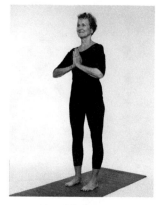

Mountain Pose, on the mat

BENEFITS: PHYSICAL
- Encourages spine to extend and align
- Activates and strengthens arches of feet, ankles, knees, and thighs
- Tones muscles of hips, abdomen, and buttocks
- Opens and expands chest and shoulders
- Improves posture

BENEFITS: MENTAL
- Provides stability and balance
- Improves concentration and focus

EYE FOCUS
- Forward
- Low seam

COUNTERPOSE
- None

Putting it all together: Once you find your level of flexibility, push down onto the three press points in your feet and engage the muscles of your legs and buttocks. Pressing your palms down onto your thighs or together gently or firmly, engage your abdominal muscles and lift your sternum. Bring your chin parallel to the ground and lift the crown of your head to lengthen your spine and the back of your neck. Rest your tongue on the roof of your mouth with the tip against the back of your front teeth. Draw your shoulders back and down. Gaze forward, keeping your head in line with your torso, or look down to the low seam.

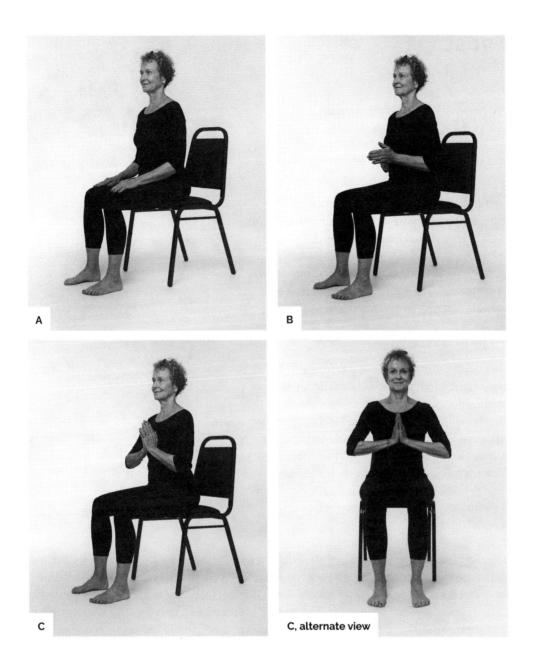

A

B

C

C, alternate view

Tips: Sitting Mountain is our foundation pose. It is the posture we start with and come back to in every chair-yoga practice, providing grounding and centering for body, mind, and spirit. Come into Sitting Mountain any time throughout the day, engaging the lower-body muscles and relaxing the upper body, reminding yourself to sit *up* on your chair for active sitting and good postural alignment.

Other options for the hands include bringing the backs of your hands onto your thighs, facing your palms up, and adding hand gestures such as Jnana Mudra or Chin Mudra (see pages 207–8).

PIGEON POSE

(Kapotasana)

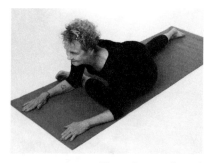

Pigeon Pose, on the mat

Begin in Sitting Mountain.

LOWER BODY: Keeping your right leg in Sitting Mountain, push down onto the three press points in your right foot. Choose to either:

A. Turn your left foot onto its outside edge, little-toe side down, then move it next to the inside of your right foot;

B. Cross your left ankle over your right ankle and flex your left foot; or

C. Raise your left leg up, keeping your knee bent, and cross it over your right thigh just above the knee, flexing your foot and allowing your left knee to open out to the side.

UPPER BODY: Choose to either:

A. Place your left hand, palm down, on the inside of your left thigh and your right hand, palm down, on the top of your right thigh; hinge forward slightly from your hips;

B. Place your left hand, palm down, on the inside of your left thigh and your right hand, palm down, on top of your right thigh; hinge farther forward from your hips; or

C. Gently rest your left hand, palm down, on the inside of your left knee or thigh and clasp your right hand around the inside of your left ankle; hinge farther forward from your hips as available.

BENEFITS: PHYSICAL
- Opens hip flexors, thighs, and chest
- Lengthens spine
- Improves digestion and circulation

BENEFITS: MENTAL
- Develops focus
- Reduces stress
- Enhances calm

EYE FOCUS
- Forward
- Low seam

COUNTERPOSES
- Backbends

Putting it all together: Once you find your level of flexibility, engage your leg muscles from the feet up into the core of your pelvis and encourage your left hip to open out to the side. Lift your sternum and hinge forward from your hips as far as available (no more than forty-five degrees). Draw your shoulders back and down, expand your chest, lift your chin slightly, and gently press your left thigh to open farther, keeping your spine lengthened. Gaze forward or down to the low seam. Return to Sitting Mountain and repeat on the other side.

Tips: The forward-folding aspects of this version of Pigeon Pose (also known as One-Legged Pigeon) can bring a sense of calm to the nervous system while opening the hips. When using your hands to help raise your leg in option C, make sure you hinge forward from your hips to keep your spine safe. If you have any bone loss, keep your torso lengthened to avoid rounding your spine. If you need to make space for the belly, you can slide the stable leg forward as needed, keeping the sole of the foot flat and the three press points engaged. For a more restorative variation, sometimes known as Resting or Sleeping Pigeon, place a soft prop on your lap once your lower body is set up, and fold your torso over in the same way as Child's Pose. For a more energizing variation, see King Pigeon Pose (page 132).

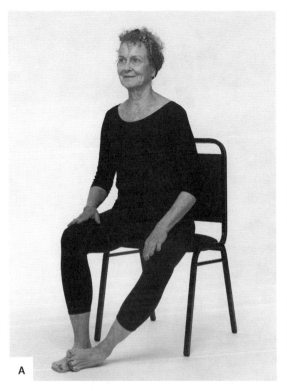

A

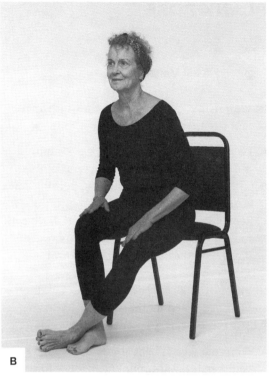

B

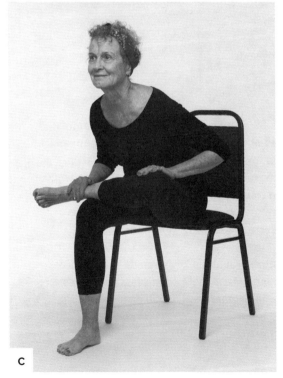

C

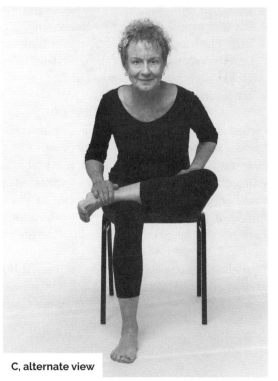

C, alternate view

PLANK POSE

(Phalakasana)

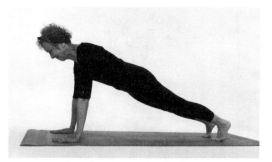

Plank Pose, on the mat

Begin in Sitting Mountain.

LOWER BODY: With your legs hip-width apart, choose to either:

A. Keep the soles of your feet on the ground, pushing down onto the three press points;
B. Come onto the balls of both feet, pushing down onto the two press points; or
C. Remaining on the balls of your feet, move both feet back toward the chair up to six inches, as available, pushing down onto the two press points.

UPPER BODY: Place the heels of your hands on your thighs and flex your hands at the wrists, palms facing forward, fingers spread wide. Choose to either:

A. Keep your elbows bent and press through the heels of your hands toward your knees; hinge forward slightly from your hips;
B. Lift your hands up to chest height, keeping your elbows bent; hinge farther forward from your hips; or
C. Lengthen your arms out at shoulder height, keeping your elbows slightly bent, or straighten them as available; hinge farther forward from your hips as available.

BENEFITS: PHYSICAL
- Strengthens arms, wrists, and spine
- Tones abdominal and core muscles
- Fosters good postural alignment

BENEFITS: MENTAL
- Develops confidence

EYE FOCUS
- Forward

COUNTERPOSE
- Sitting Mountain

Putting it all together: Once you find your level of flexibility, engage your thigh and abdominal muscles by pushing the press points in your feet down onto the ground. Lift your sternum and hinge forward from your hips as far as available (no more than forty-five degrees) and keep your spine lengthened. As available, either stretch or visualize a dynamic stretch through your hands as you press them against an imaginary wall in front of you. Draw your shoulders back and down, and expand your chest. Gaze forward, keeping your head in line with your torso and your neck lengthened. Come out of the pose and return to Sitting Mountain.

Tips: Also known as Four-Limbed Staff Pose, this posture provides a key strengthening aspect to every Sun Salutation. Hold Plank Pose for three breaths if available, then press your arms back and forth dynamically, doing push-ups against an imaginary wall while on a chair.

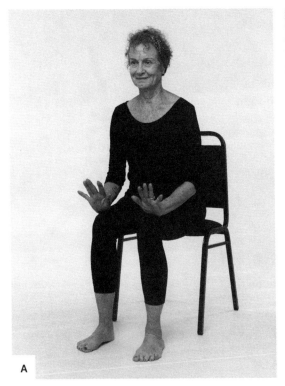

A

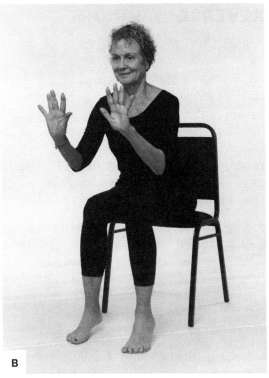

B

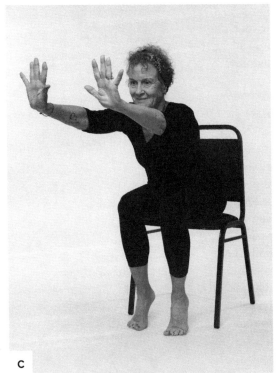

C

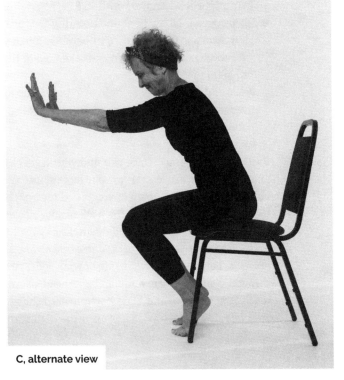

C, alternate view

REVERSE WARRIOR
(Viparita Virabhadrasana)

Begin in Sitting Mountain. Turn and face the right side of the chair and reestablish Sitting Mountain. Keep your right buttock on the chair; your left buttock may extend off the chair as needed, keeping both sit bones on the chair.

LOWER BODY: With your right leg in Sitting Mountain, press down onto the three press points in your right foot. Choose to either:

A. Bring your left leg into a V-shaped position;
B. Bring your left leg into an L-shaped position; or
C. Bring your left leg into an extended position, as available; turn your left foot to face forward with the sole flat on the ground, adjusting your buttocks on the chair as needed.

UPPER BODY: Choose to either:

A. Bend your right elbow so that your forearm and upper arm are at a right angle and your palm is facing inward; bring your left hand to your hip;
B. Keeping your elbow bent and pointing forward, lift your right arm and place your right hand on top of your head, extend your left arm down and take hold of the chair seat or leg on the left; or
C. Raise and lengthen your right arm to arch up and overhead; place your left hand on your left leg, if it is extended.

Putting it all together: Once you find your level of flexibility, engage your leg muscles from your feet up into the core of your pelvis. Lift the crown of your head toward the ceiling to lengthen your spine and the back of your neck as you relax your shoulders back and down. Lean your torso back, draw your right shoulder back, and engage your abdominal muscles. Lengthen the right side of your body, stretching through your right arm and hand overhead, as available; reach your left arm and hand down toward the ground on your left side. Gaze forward or up at the high seam. To come

(CONTINUED ON NEXT SPREAD)

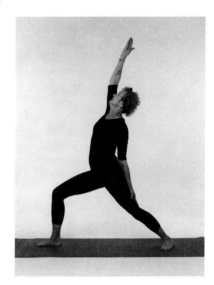

Reverse Warrior, on the mat

BENEFITS: PHYSICAL
- Strengthens and stretches legs, groin, hips, waist, side body, shoulders, arms, and neck
- Enhances flexibility in groin, spine, and chest
- Stimulates circulation
- Can help relieve low back pain
- Improves balance
- Reduces fatigue

BENEFITS: MENTAL
- Calms the mind
- Boosts confidence

EYE FOCUS
- Forward
- High seam

COUNTERPOSES
- Humble Warrior
- Warrior II

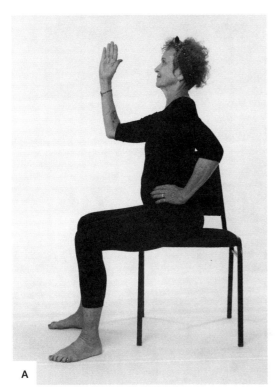

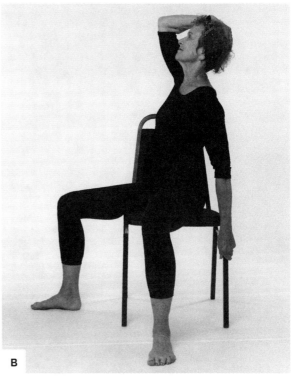

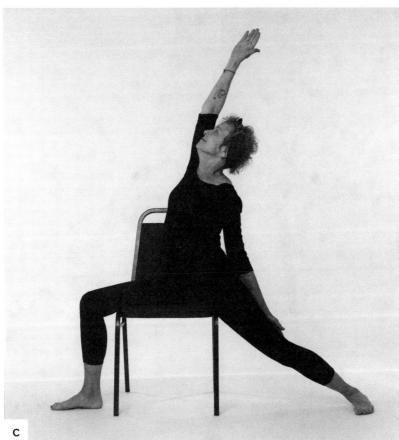

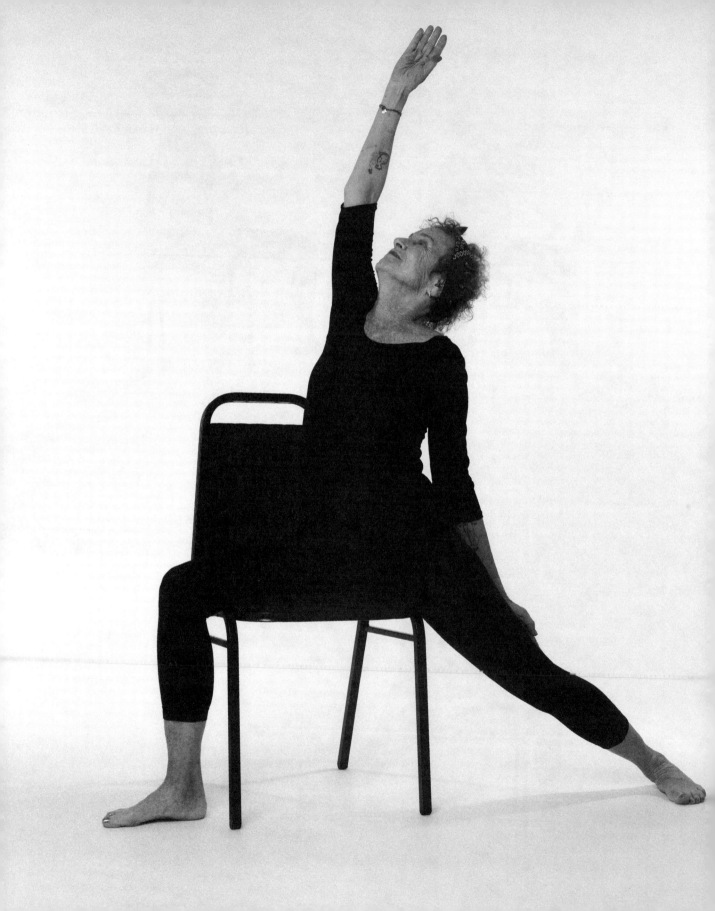

out of the pose, return to Sitting Mountain on the right side of the chair before moving to the front of the chair into Sitting Mountain. Repeat on the other side.

Tips: If you are lifting and raising an arm overhead, remember to soften and relax your shoulder to avoid strain. If you feel faint, lightheaded, or dizzy when raising an arm, keep your head level, looking forward with your eyes, not up. Also known as Peaceful Warrior, Reverse Warrior can be set up on the front of the chair as an alternative, following the lower-body instructions for Warrior II (page 178). In a chair with arms, follow the lower-body options in Squat Pose (page 158)—Sitting Mountain legs, V-shaped legs, and L-shaped legs.

Reverse Warrior (option C, alternative view)

REVOLVED CHAIR POSE

(Parivritta Utkatasana)

Begin in Sitting Mountain.

LOWER BODY: With your legs hip-width apart, choose to either:

A. Keep the soles of your feet on the ground, pushing down onto the three press points;

B. Come onto the balls of both feet, pushing down onto the two press points; or

C. Remaining on the balls of both feet, move both feet back up to six inches, pushing down onto the two press points.

UPPER BODY: Bring your palms together, pressing your thumbs onto your sternum, and lift your elbows. Choose to either:

A. Turn your torso to the left;

B. Turn your torso farther to the left, lowering your right elbow onto your right thigh as available; or

C. Turn your torso even farther to the left and extend your right elbow down onto your left thigh or to the outside of your left thigh as available.

Putting it all together: Once you find your level of flexibility, push down onto the press points in your feet and engage the muscles of your legs and buttocks. With your palms pressed together at your sternum, lift the crown of your head to lengthen your spine and the back of your neck and draw your shoulders back and down. Extend and lengthen your torso to the left, drawing your left shoulder back and keeping your head in line with your torso. Lift your left elbow up from the shoulder, as available, with your right elbow extending down toward or onto your thigh. Gaze forward or up to the high seam, or turn to look over your left shoulder. Return to Sitting Mountain and repeat on the other side.

Tips: Gently rotating the spine in Revolved Chair Pose and other twisting postures offers a safe and effective way to stretch the back and release tightness in the spine. If you need to make space for the belly, you can widen your legs into a V-shaped or L-shaped position.

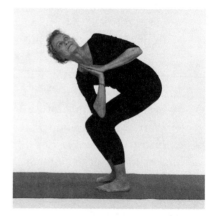

Revolved Chair Pose, on the mat

BENEFITS: PHYSICAL
- Increases spinal and abdominal flexibility
- Strengthens feet, ankles, calves, knees, thighs, buttocks, arms, and hands
- Opens chest and shoulders
- Stimulates digestion and circulation
- May alleviate menstrual symptoms

BENEFITS: MENTAL
- Helps relieve stress and lift mood
- Builds confidence

EYE FOCUS
- Forward
- High seam
- Over shoulder

COUNTERPOSE
- Sitting Mountain

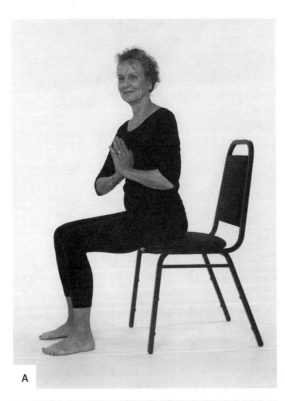

A

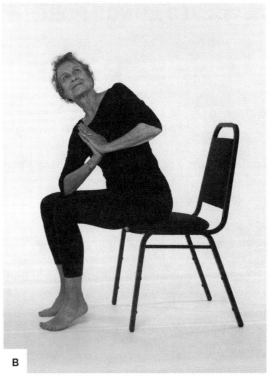

B

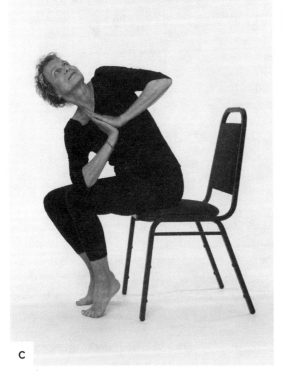

C

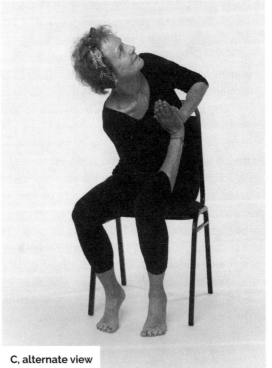

C, alternate view

REVOLVED LUNGE POSE

(Parivritta Ashta Chandrasana)

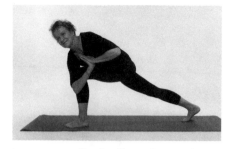

Revolved Lunge Pose, on the mat

Begin in Sitting Mountain. Turn and face the left side of the chair and reestablish Sitting Mountain. Keep your left buttock on the chair; your right buttock may extend off the chair as needed, keeping both sit bones on the chair.

LOWER BODY: Keep your left leg in Sitting Mountain, pushing down onto the three press points in your foot. To position the right leg, choose to either:

A. Bring your right leg into a V-shaped position;
B. Bring your right leg into an L-shaped position; or
C. Bring your right leg into an extended position, as available; come onto the ball of your right foot, adjusting your buttocks on the chair as needed.

UPPER BODY: Choose to either:

A. Place your hands, palms down, on your thighs; turn your torso to the left, keeping your head in line with your torso;
B. Bring your palms together, press your thumbs onto your sternum, and turn your torso farther to the left; turn your head so that it is in line with your torso; or
C. Bring your palms together, press your thumbs onto your sternum, and turn your torso even farther to the left, extending your right elbow down onto the left thigh or to the outside of your left thigh, as available; turn your head in line with your torso.

Putting it all together: Once you find your level of flexibility, press down onto the press points in your feet and engage your legs and buttocks. With your palms on your thighs or pressed together at your sternum, lift the crown of your head to lengthen your spine, and draw your shoulders back and down. Extend and lengthen your torso, and turn to the left, drawing your left shoulder back and keeping your head in line with your torso. With palms pressed together, lift your left elbow up, as available, and extend your right elbow down toward, onto, or outside your left thigh. Gaze forward or up to the high seam, or turn to look over your left shoulder. To come out of the pose, return to Sitting Mountain on the left side of the chair before moving to the front of the chair into Sitting Mountain. Repeat on the other side.

Tips: Bringing the palms together in front of the chest in Anjali Mudra and engaging the arm and hand muscles helps augment core strength in postures such as Revolved Lunge Pose. For related poses, see High Lunge Pose (page 124) and Lunge Pose (page 140).

BENEFITS: PHYSICAL
- Strengthens and tones feet, ankles, and leg muscles
- Increases pelvic floor and core muscle strength
- Expands chest
- Increases spinal flexibility
- Massages and tones abdominal organs and muscles
- Stimulates digestion and circulation
- Improves balance and coordination

BENEFITS: MENTAL
- Helps relieve stress and lift mood

EYE FOCUS
- Forward
- High seam
- Over shoulder

COUNTERPOSE
- Sitting Mountain

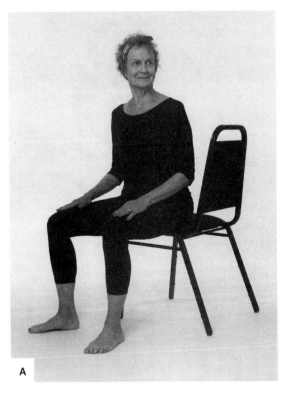

A

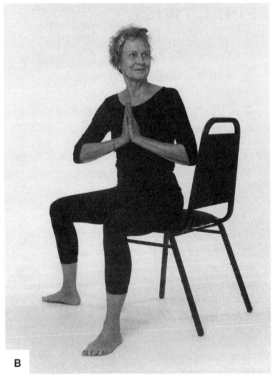

B

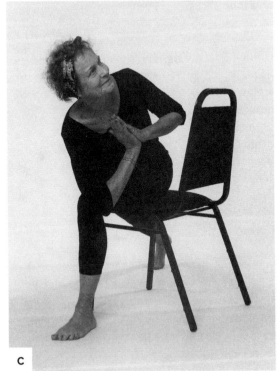

C

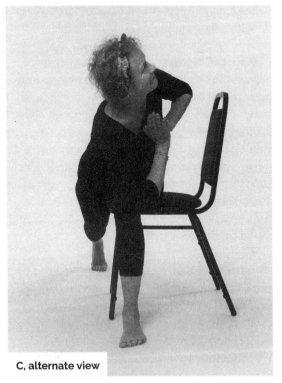

C, alternate view

SPINAL TWIST

(Parivritta Sukhasana)

Begin in Sitting Mountain.

LOWER BODY: Keep your legs in Sitting Mountain, pushing down onto the three press points in your feet.

UPPER BODY: Lift the crown of your head toward the ceiling to lengthen the neck and spine. Choose to either:

A. Rotate your torso slightly to the right; place your right hand on your right thigh, palm down, bringing the heel of your hand in close to your body; place your left hand in front of your right hand, palm down;

B. Rotating your torso farther to the right, bring your right hand to hold on to the right side of the chair seat; place your left hand on the outside of your right thigh; or

C. Rotating farther to the right, bring your right hand behind your back, flex your right wrist, and place your right palm flat on the chair seat with your fingers pointing away from your buttocks; place your left hand on the outside of your right thigh or knee, straightening your arm and extending your hand down.

Putting it all together: Once you find your level of flexibility, engage your leg and buttock muscles by pushing the three press points in both feet down onto the ground. Draw your shoulders back and down, expanding your chest. Continue to lift the crown of your head toward the ceiling and lengthen your spine as you rotate your torso or visualize doing this. Engage your upper-body muscles by either pressing your hands down onto your body or visualizing pressing them down. Gaze forward or over your right shoulder, rotating your neck, as available. Return to Sitting Mountain and repeat on the other side.

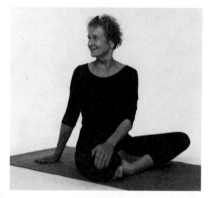

Spinal Twist, on the mat

BENEFITS: PHYSICAL
- Increases spinal and abdominal flexibility
- Lengthens and strengthens spine, shoulders, and hips
- Oxygenates internal organs
- Alleviates backache, neck injury, and sciatica
- Stimulates digestion and circulation
- Relieves menstrual symptoms

BENEFITS: MENTAL
- Helps relieve stress and lift mood

EYE FOCUS
- Forward
- Over shoulder

COUNTERPOSES
- Sitting Mountain
- Forward Fold

Tips: In this version of Spinal Twist, the head turns in the same direction as the torso. To release the spine further, turn your head to face in the opposite direction. For a variation called Ardha Matsyendrasana, bring your legs and feet together with your knees in line with your navel, cross your legs at the ankles or knees, then squeeze your legs together to further engage the lower-body muscles. Before coming into a Spinal Twist, be sure to lengthen your spine and neck to keep your back safe. When rotating your torso, soften and relax your shoulders and jaw. Remember to focus on lengthening your spine more than deepening the twist, especially if you have any back challenges. Avoid using your arms or hands to pull your body too deep into the twist.

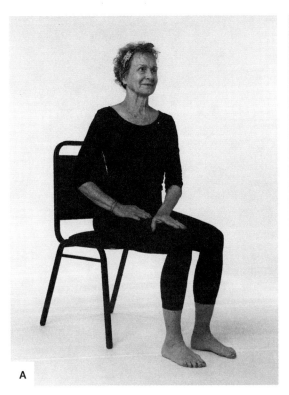

A

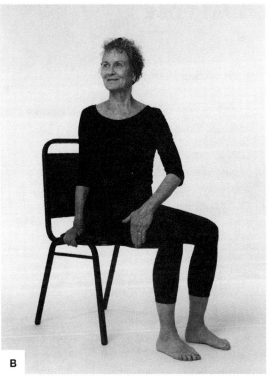

B

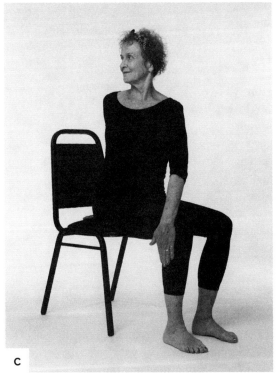

C

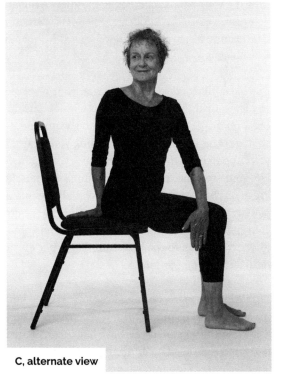

C, alternate view

SQUAT POSE

(Malasana)

Begin in Sitting Mountain.

LOWER BODY: Pushing down onto the three press points in your feet, choose to either:

A. Leave your legs in Sitting Mountain;
B. Bring your legs into a V-shaped position, pointing your toes out in the same direction as your knees; or
C. Bring both legs into a wider V-shaped position or an L-shaped position, pointing your toes out in the same direction as your knees.

UPPER BODY: Bring your palms together in Anjali Mudra and choose to either:

A. Bring your palms together at abdomen level, fingers pointing forward, and hinge forward slightly from your hips;
B. Bring your palms together at chest level, fingers pointing up, and hinge farther forward from your hips; or
C. Bring your hands together at chest level, fingers pointing up, and place the knuckles of your thumbs onto your sternum; hinge even farther forward from your hips as available.

Putting it all together: Once you find your level of flexibility, engage your thigh and buttock muscles by pushing the three press points in both feet down onto the ground. Draw your shoulders back and down, expanding your chest. Engage your upper-body muscles by pressing your palms together. Lift your sternum, engage your abdominal muscles, and hinge forward from your hips as available, going as far as placing your elbows inside your knees. Lift the crown of your head to lengthen your torso, neck, and spine, and gaze forward or down to the low seam. Come out of the pose and return to Sitting Mountain.

Tips: Also known as Garland Pose, Squat Pose builds core as well as spinal strength, benefiting both balance and posture. If you have any bone loss, keep your torso lengthened to avoid rounding your spine. If you have lower back issues, visualize hinging forward instead. If you feel faint, lightheaded, or dizzy and this pose does not feel comfortable, keep your head above your heart, moving into whatever level of flexibility feels doable and visualizing the rest.

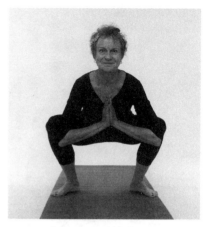

Squat Pose, on the mat

BENEFITS: PHYSICAL
- Stretches and strengthens shoulders, chest, hips, and back
- Increases pelvic floor and core muscle strength
- Stimulates digestion and circulation
- Relieves back pain
- Improves balance and posture

BENEFITS: MENTAL
- Develops concentration and focus

EYE FOCUS
- Forward
- Low seam

COUNTERPOSE
- Sitting Mountain

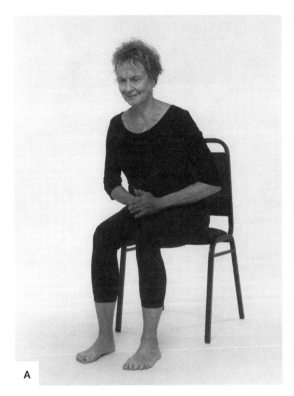

A

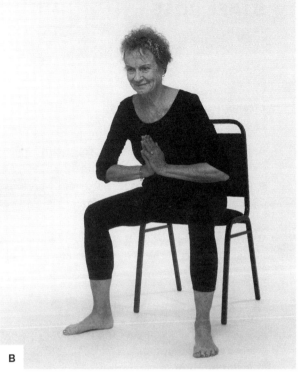

B

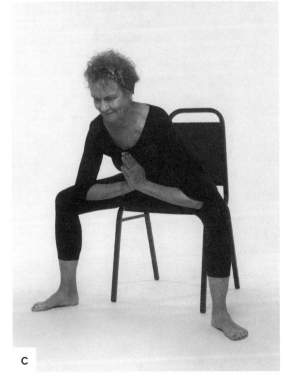

C

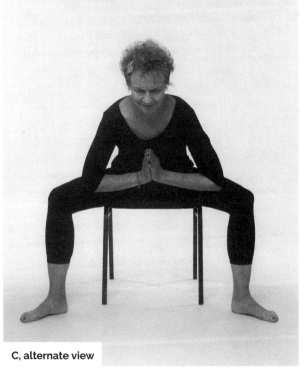

C, alternate view

STAFF POSE

(Dandasana)

Begin in Sitting Mountain.

LOWER BODY: With your legs hip-width apart, choose to either:

A. Keep the soles of your feet on the ground, pushing down onto the three press points;
B. Extend your lower legs forward with your knees bent and the soles of your feet on the ground, pushing down onto the three press points; or
C. Bring your legs together and straighten them, as available; flex your feet at the ankles, pressing your heels onto the ground.

UPPER BODY: Choose to either:

A. Place your hands on your thighs, palms down, bringing the heels of your hands in close to your body, elbows pointing back;
B. Place the heels of your hands on either side of the chair seat, fingers extending down or out to the side; or
C. Bring your hands behind your back, flex your wrists, and place your palms flat on the chair seat with your fingers pointing toward your buttocks.

Putting it all together: Once you find your level of flexibility, engage your leg and abdominal muscles from the feet up into the core of your pelvis. Draw your shoulders back and down, bringing your shoulder blades toward each other. Engage your arm and upper-body muscles by either pressing your hands down or visualizing pressing them down. Lift your sternum and the crown of your head toward the ceiling to lengthen your torso, neck, and spine; continue to draw your shoulders back and down; and gaze forward. Come out of the pose and return to Sitting Mountain.

Tip: Staff Pose increases body awareness and core strength and, like Sitting Mountain, it helps to enhance and maintain good posture.

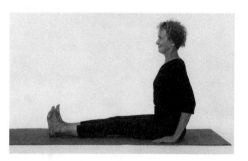

Eight-Limbed Pose, on the mat

BENEFITS: PHYSICAL
- Improves posture and balance
- Strengthens feet, legs, abdomen, and arms
- Lengthens and stretches spine and strengthens back muscles
- Opens and stretches shoulders and chest
- Tones abdominal and core muscles
- Improves posture
- Stimulates circulation
- Relieves fatigue

BENEFITS: MENTAL
- Improves focus
- Helps calm and stabilize the mind
- Reduces stress

EYE FOCUS
- Forward

COUNTERPOSES
- Sitting Mountain
- Forward Fold

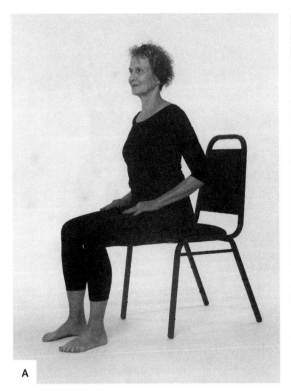

A

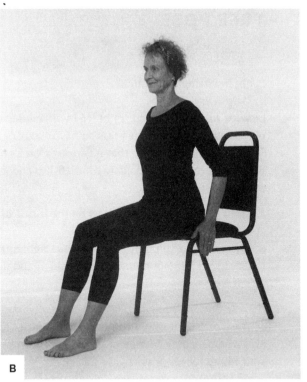

B

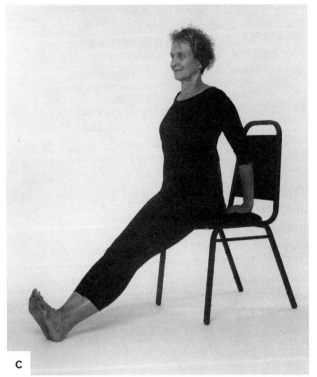

C

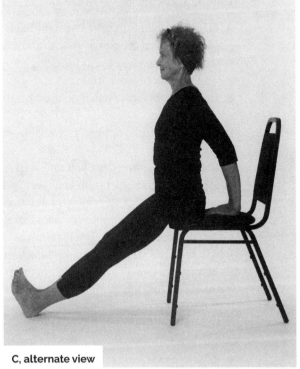

C, alternate view

TREE POSE

(Vrikshasana)

Begin in Sitting Mountain.

LOWER BODY: With your right leg in Sitting Mountain, push down onto the three press points in your right foot. Turn your left foot out so that it is resting on its outer edge, little-toe side down, and allow your left hip and knee to fall open. Choose to either:

A. Move your left foot over to rest on the inside of your right foot;
B. Cross and flex your left foot over your right ankle; or
C. Place your left foot onto your right thigh and flex your left foot.

Note: In option C, you can use your hands to assist raising your leg onto your thigh; be sure to hinge forward from your hips when bending down to keep your spine safe, and flex your raised foot to protect your knee joint.

UPPER BODY: Choose to either:

A. Place your hands in your lap, right hand on top of left, palms up; join the tips of your thumbs together and place the outsides of your little fingers against your lower abdomen in Dhyana Mudra;
B. Bring your palms together at chest height in Anjali Mudra; or
C. Raise your arms overhead as available, palms together.

Putting it all together: Once you find your level of flexibility, engage your leg muscles from your feet up into the core of your pelvis. Lift your sternum and draw your shoulders back and down, lengthening your torso and spine. Engage your upper-body muscles and either stretch or visualize your hands and arms stretching up, keeping your body vertical. Gaze forward, down to the low seam, or up to the high seam. Return to Sitting Mountain and repeat on the other side.

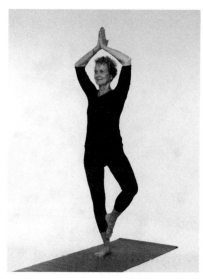

Tree Pose, on the mat

BENEFITS: PHYSICAL
- Improves balance, coordination, and core strength
- Strengthens arches, ankles, calves, and thighs
- Lengthens spine
- Opens shoulders, chest, thighs, and hips
- Improves circulation

BENEFITS: MENTAL
- Cultivates focus and alertness
- Fosters mental clarity
- Builds confidence

EYE FOCUS
- Forward
- Low seam
- High seam

COUNTERPOSE
- Sitting Mountain

(CONTINUED ON NEXT SPREAD)

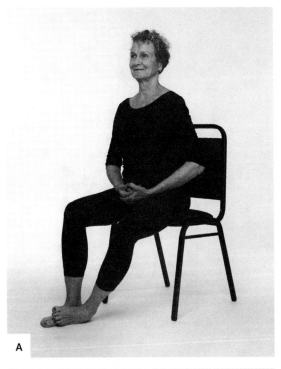

A

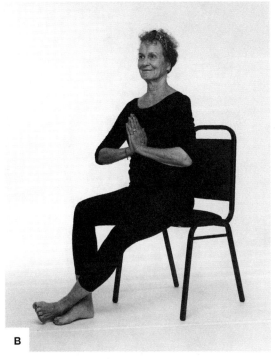

B

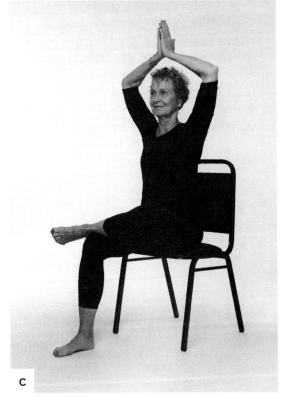

C

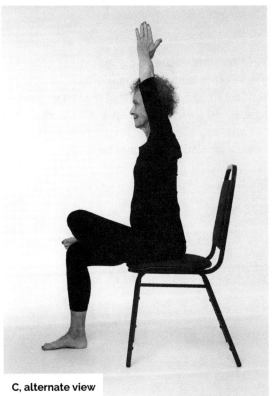

C, alternate view

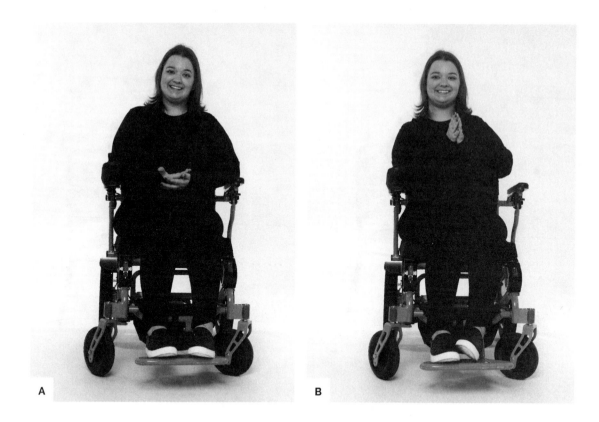

A   B

Tips: Tree Pose invites many options for both the lower and upper body. See pages 37–38 for examples of this posture in even more levels of flexibility as well as mix-and-match options! Also shown here are three options for Tree Pose on a wheelchair. Visualize the tree of your choice when doing this pose. If you are lifting and raising your arms overhead, remember to soften and relax your shoulders to avoid strain. If you feel faint, lightheaded, or dizzy when raising your arms, keep your head level, looking forward with your eyes, not up.

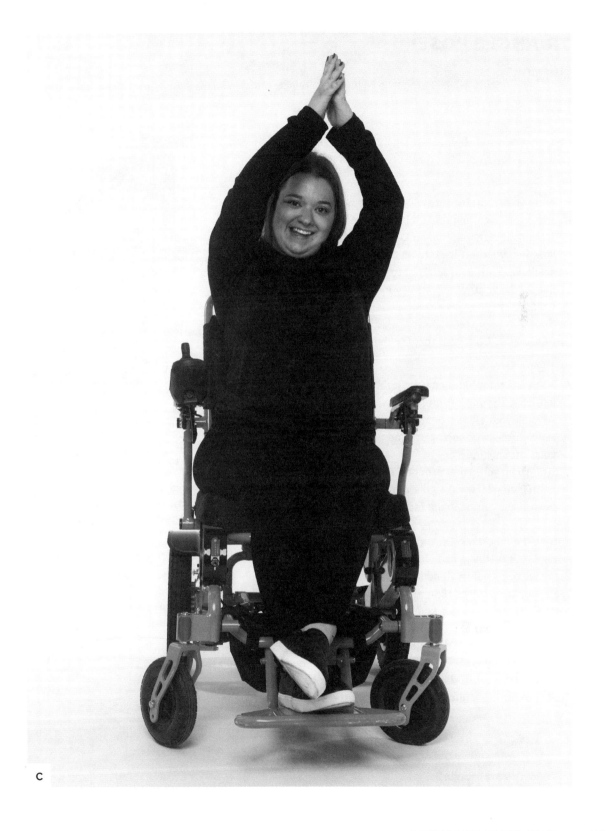

C

TRIANGLE POSE

(Trikonasana)

Begin in Sitting Mountain.

LOWER BODY: With your left leg in Sitting Mountain position, push down onto the three press points in the left foot. Choose to either:

A. Bring your right leg into a V-shaped position;
B. Bring your right leg into an L-shaped position; or
C. Bring your right leg into an L-shaped position and lengthen your left leg into an extended position, as available. Turn your left foot to face forward with the sole flat on the ground, adjusting your buttocks on the chair as needed.

UPPER BODY: Lean your torso to the right and choose to either:

A. Rest your right hand on your right thigh and bring your left hand to your left hip;
B. Keeping your elbows bent, rest your right forearm on your right thigh, palm facing up, and place your left hand onto your left shoulder; or
C. Straighten your right arm down inside your right leg, palm facing forward, and straighten your left arm up toward the ceiling, palm facing forward.

Putting it all together: Once you find your level of flexibility, engage your feet, leg, and abdominal muscles by pushing the three press points in both feet down onto the ground. Lean your torso to the right and draw your left shoulder back. Engage your upper-body muscles by either stretching or visualizing your arms and hands stretching upward and downward in opposite directions, lengthening both the front and left side of your body, as available. Lengthen your neck by dipping your chin slightly and gaze up, forward, or down. Return to Sitting Mountain and repeat on the other side.

(CONTINUED ON NEXT SPREAD)

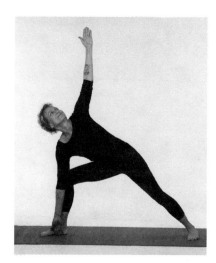

Triangle Pose, on the mat

BENEFITS: PHYSICAL
- Stabilizes and strengthens legs and core muscles
- Strengthens and stretches arches, feet, ankles, calves, hamstrings, and groin
- Lengthens the spine
- Tones arms
- Opens throat, chest, rib cage, shoulders, and hips
- Increases muscular stamina
- Improves circulation and digestion

BENEFITS: MENTAL
- Builds focus
- Relieves stress
- Fosters willpower and determination
- Stimulates attention and concentration

EYE FOCUS
- Upward
- Forward
- Downward

COUNTERPOSES
- Sitting Mountain
- Warrior II

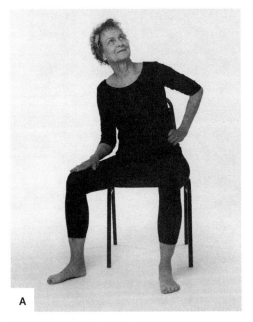

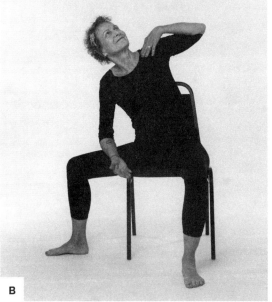

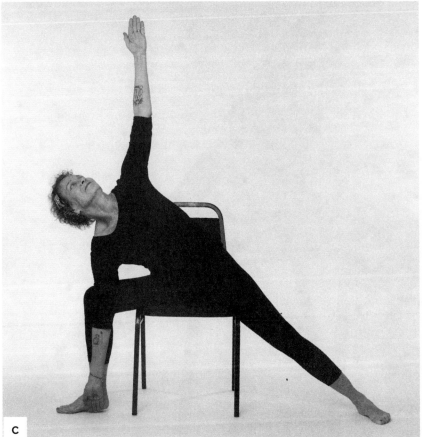

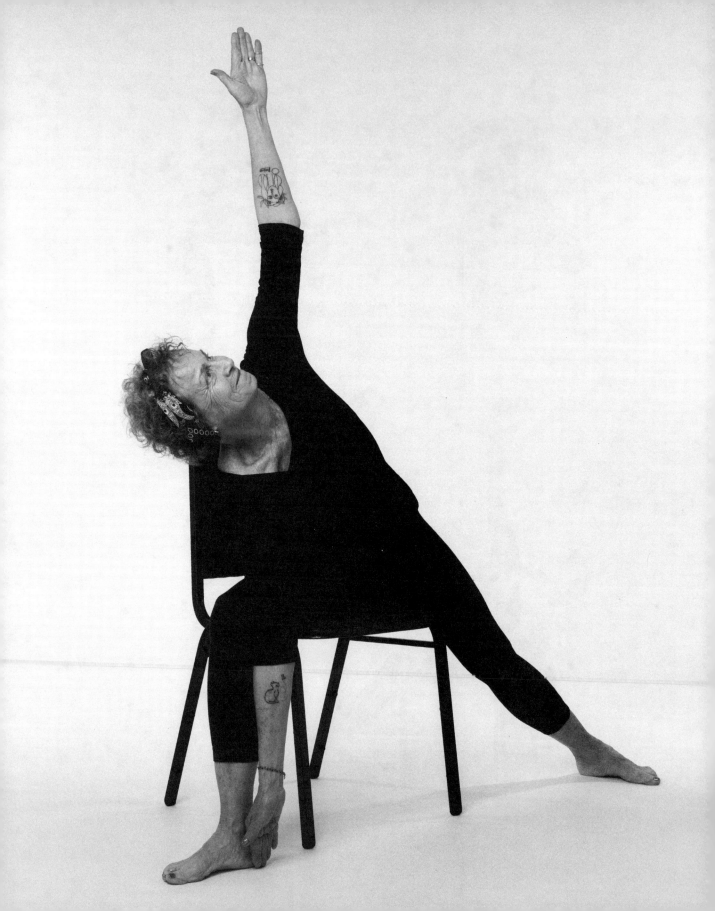

Tips: With the front knee bent, this pose is also known as Extended Triangle Pose (Utthita Trikonasana). Triangle Pose can also be set up from the side of the chair following the lower-body instructions for Warrior I (page 174). If you are using a chair with arms, for the lower body, choose options A or B, or keep your legs in Sitting Mountain; see the lower-body instructions for Squat Pose (page 158).

If you are lifting an arm overhead, remember to soften and relax your shoulder to avoid strain. If you feel faint, lightheaded, or dizzy when raising an arm, keep your head level, looking forward with your eyes and not up.

Triangle Pose (option C, alternative view)

UPWARD SALUTE

(Urdhva Hastasana)

Begin in Sitting Mountain.

LOWER BODY: Keep your legs in Sitting Mountain, pushing down onto the three press points in your feet.

UPPER BODY: Keeping your arms shoulder-width apart, turn your palms to face each other. Choose to either:

A. Bend your elbows at waist height, in close to your body;
B. Keeping your elbows bent, lift your hands to chest or head height; or
C. Straighten your arms up toward the ceiling, as available.

Putting it all together: Once you find your level of flexibility, engage your leg, buttock, and abdominal muscles by pushing the three press points in both feet down onto the ground. Engage your upper-body muscles by lifting your sternum, and either stretch or visualize stretching your arms and hands long. Draw your shoulders back and down to lengthen your torso and spine. Lift the crown of your head up toward the ceiling. Gaze forward or up to the high seam. Come out of the pose and return to Sitting Mountain.

Tips: Upward Salute is the first pose you move into in a Sun Salutation, raising the arms to greet the sun following Sitting Mountain. Once you come into this pose, you can arch your back slightly, as available, to energize the body and the mind. If you are lifting and raising your arms overhead, remember to soften and relax your shoulders to avoid strain. If you feel faint, lightheaded, or dizzy when raising your arms, keep your head level, looking forward with your eyes, not up.

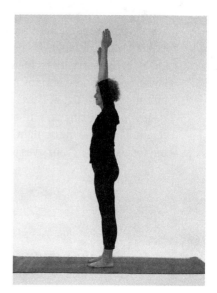

Upward Salute, on the mat

BENEFITS: PHYSICAL
- Strengthens shoulders, armpits, arms, and hands
- Lengthens abdomen
- Massages internal organs
- Improves digestion

BENEFITS: MENTAL
- Lifts mood
- Calms the mind

EYE FOCUS
- Forward
- High seam

COUNTERPOSE
- Forward Fold

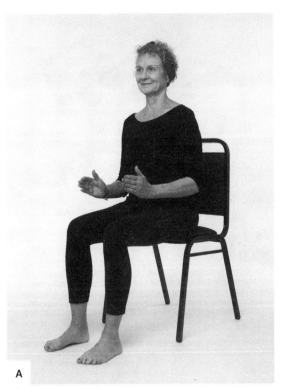

A

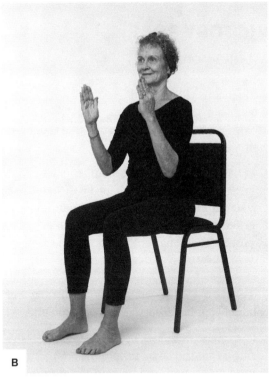

B

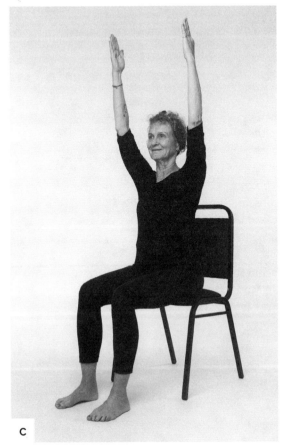

C

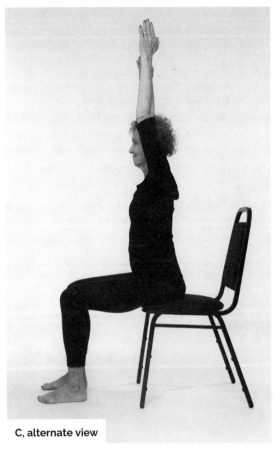

C, alternate view

VICTORY POSE

(Utkata Konasana)

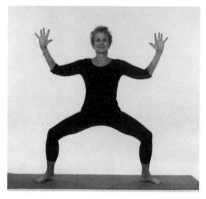

Victory Pose, on the mat

Begin in Sitting Mountain.

LOWER BODY: Pushing down onto the three press points in your feet, choose to either:

A. Leave your legs in Sitting Mountain;
B. Bring your legs into a V-shaped position, pointing your toes out in the same direction as your knees; or
C. Bring your legs into a wider V-shaped or an L-shaped position, pointing your toes out in the same direction as your knees.

UPPER BODY: Bring your arms by your sides and face the palms of your hands forward. Choose to either:

A. Keep your arms down by your sides and stretch your fingers out and down toward the ground;
B. Bend your elbows and lift your hands to shoulder height, stretching your fingers out and up as available; or
C. Bend your elbows at shoulder height and, as available, lift your arms into right angles and stretch your fingers out and up.

Putting it all together: Once you find your level of flexibility, engage the muscles of your legs, buttocks, and abdomen by pushing the three press points in both feet down onto the ground. Lift your sternum and draw your shoulders back and down. Lift the crown of your head toward the ceiling, lengthening your neck and spine. Engage your upper-body muscles and spread and stretch your fingers and thumbs, or visualize doing this. Gaze forward or down to the low seam. Come out of the pose and return to Sitting Mountain.

Tips: You can raise your arms and stretch your fingers and thumbs wide into "cactus arms," or choose a hand gesture, such as Jnana Mudra or Chin Mudra (see pages 207–8), to direct and strengthen physical and mental energy. This posture is also known as Goddess Pose (Deviasana).

BENEFITS: PHYSICAL
- Aligns spine and improves posture
- Expands chest
- Stretches arms and side body
- Tones abdominal and buttock muscles
- Strengthens arches, ankles, knees, and legs
- Stimulates circulation

BENEFITS: MENTAL
- Develops attention and motivation
- Lifts mood
- Relieves stress

EYE FOCUS
- Forward
- Low seam

COUNTERPOSE
- Crescent Moon Pose

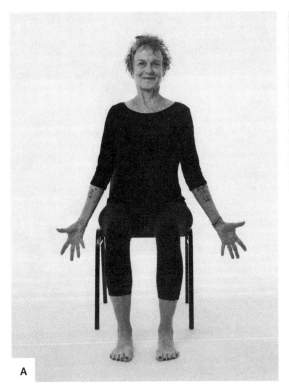

A

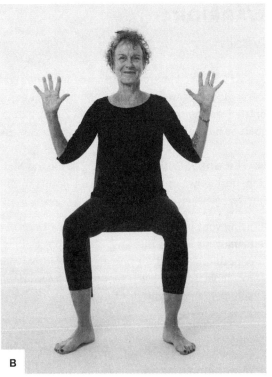

B

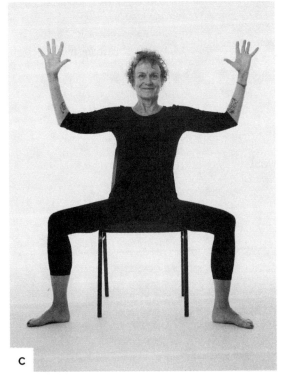

C

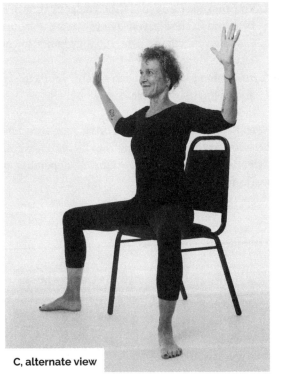

C, alternate view

WARRIOR I

(Virabhadrasana I)

Begin in Sitting Mountain. Turn and face the right side of the chair and reestablish Sitting Mountain. Keep your right buttock on the chair; your left buttock may extend off the chair as needed, keeping both sit bones on the chair.

LOWER BODY: With your right leg in Sitting Mountain position, push down onto the three press points in the right foot. Choose to either:

A. Bring your left leg into a V-shaped position;
B. Bring your left leg into an L-shaped position; or
C. Lengthen your left leg into an extended position, as available; turn your left foot to face forward with the sole flat on the ground, adjusting your buttocks on the chair as needed.

UPPER BODY: Keeping your arms shoulder-width apart, turn your palms to face each other. Choose to either:

A. Rest the outside of your hands on your thighs, elbows bent and in close to your body;
B. Keeping your elbows bent, lift your hands to chest or head height; or
C. Straighten your elbows and extend your arms as fully and as high as available.

Note: Remember that you can bring your arms anywhere between resting on your thighs to lifting them fully extended overhead next to your ears, depending on what works for you on the day.

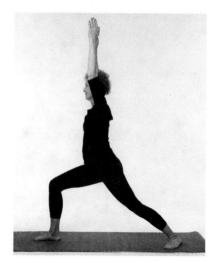

Warrior I, on the mat

BENEFITS: PHYSICAL
- Strengthens arches, ankles, knees, legs, back, and arms
- Stretches and opens arms, shoulders, psoas, and hips
- Supports knee strength and stability
- Increases pelvic floor and core muscle strength
- Expands chest
- Stimulates digestion and circulation
- Relieves sciatica and back pain
- Improves balance

BENEFITS: MENTAL
- Builds concentration and focus
- Develops attention and motivation
- Energizes mood

EYE FOCUS
- Forward
- High seam

COUNTERPOSE
- Sitting Mountain

(CONTINUED ON NEXT SPREAD)

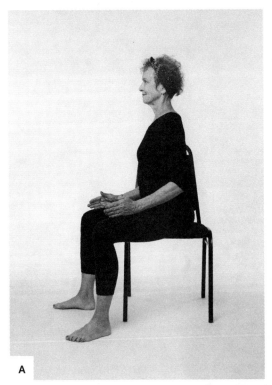

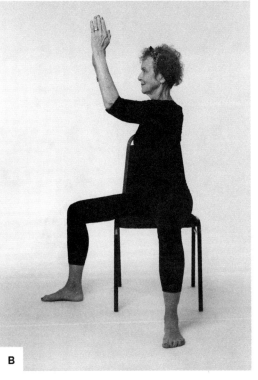

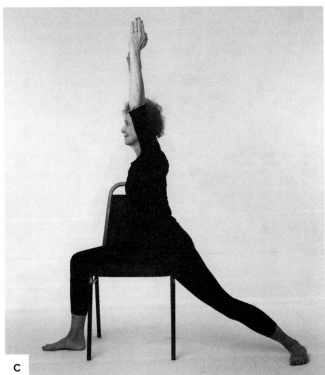

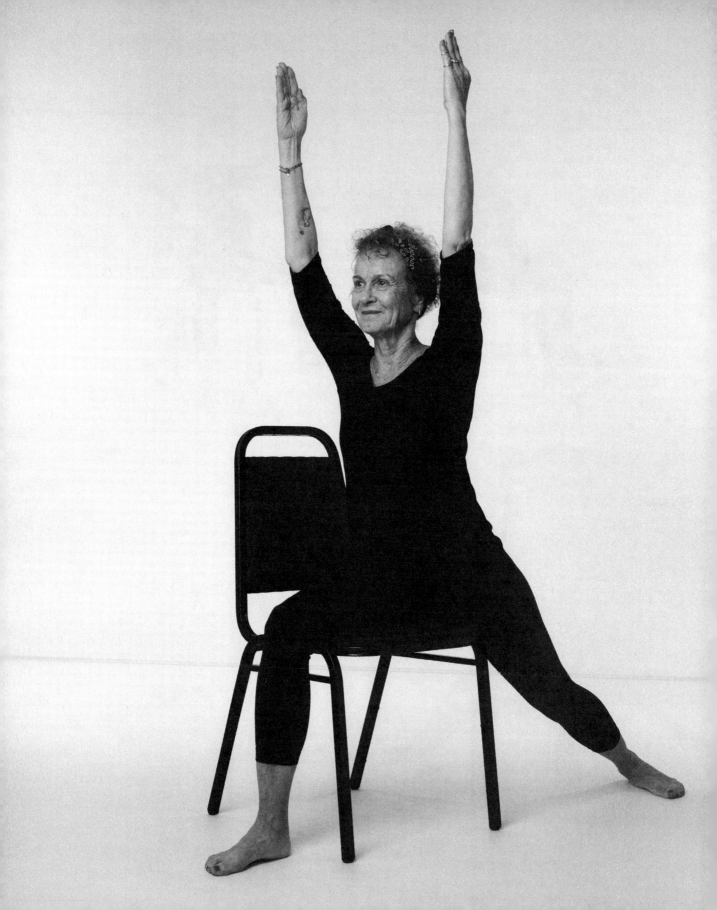

Putting it all together: Once you find your level of flexibility, engage your thigh and abdominal muscles by pushing the three press points in both feet down onto the ground. Engage your upper-body muscles by lifting your sternum and stretching your arms and hands. Draw your shoulders back and down to lengthen your torso and spine. Gaze forward or up to the high seam. To come out of the pose, return to Sitting Mountain on the right side of the chair before moving to the front of the chair into Sitting Mountain. Repeat on the other side.

Tips: Warrior I can be set up on the front of the chair as an alternative, following the lower-body instructions for Warrior II (page 178). In a chair with arms, follow the lower-body options in Squat Pose (page 158)—Sitting Mountain legs, V-shaped leg, and L-shaped leg. If you are lifting and raising your arms overhead, remember to soften and relax your shoulders to avoid strain. If you feel faint, lightheaded, or dizzy when raising your arms, keep your head level, looking forward with your eyes, not up.

Warrior I (option C, alternative view)

WARRIOR II

(Virabhadrasana II)

Begin in Sitting Mountain.

LOWER BODY: With your left leg in Sitting Mountain position, push down onto the three press points in the left foot. Keep your hips facing forward and choose to either:

A. Bring your right leg into a V-shaped position;
B. Bring your right leg into an L-shaped position; or
C. Bring your right leg into an L-shaped position and lengthen your left leg into an extended position, as available; turn your left foot to face forward with the sole flat on the ground, adjusting your buttocks on the chair as needed.

UPPER BODY: Choose to either:

A. Keep your hands in Sitting Mountain, palms resting down on your thighs;
B. Place your hands on your shoulders, lifting your bent elbows as high as available; or
C. Extend your right arm forward and your left arm back at shoulder height, reaching in opposite directions parallel to the ground, palms facing down.

Putting it all together: Once you find your level of flexibility, engage your thigh and abdominal muscles by pushing the three press points in both feet down onto the ground. Keeping your hips facing forward, engage your upper-body muscles by lifting your sternum and stretching your arms and hands in opposite directions. Draw your shoulders back and down to lengthen your torso and spine. Gaze forward with your head in line with your torso or turn your head to look over the fingertips of your extended right hand. Return to Sitting Mountain and repeat on the other side.

Tips: Warrior II can help build physical strength and stamina as well as inner resolve and resilience. It can also be set up from the side of the chair following the lower-body instructions for Warrior I (page 174). If you are using a chair with arms, for the lower body, choose either options A or B, or keep your legs in Sitting Mountain; see the lower-body instructions for Squat Pose (page 158).

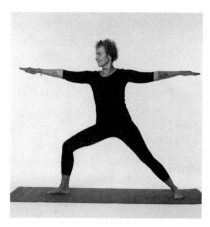

Warrior II, on the mat

BENEFITS: PHYSICAL
- Strengthens arches, ankles, knees, legs, back, and arms
- Stretches arms, shoulders, and hips
- Supports knee strength and stability
- Increases pelvic floor and core muscle strength
- Expands chest
- Stimulates digestion and circulation
- Relieves sciatica and back pain
- Improves balance

BENEFITS: MENTAL
- Builds concentration and focus
- Develops attention and motivation
- Energizes mood

EYE FOCUS
- Forward
- Over fingertips of forward extended arm

COUNTERPOSE
- Sitting Mountain

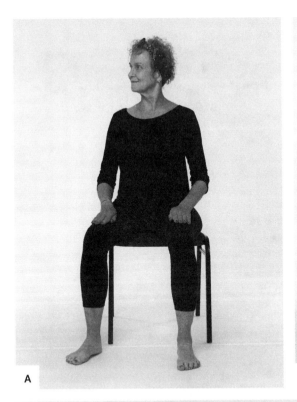

A

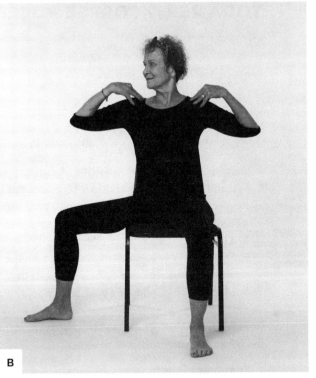

B

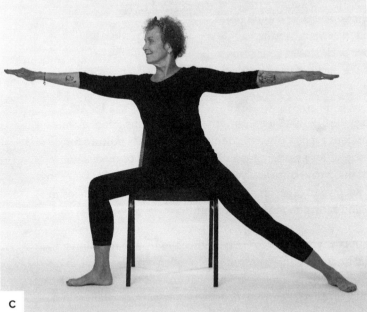

C

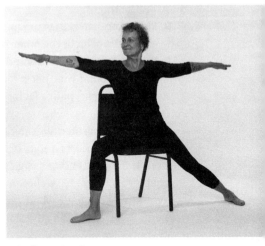

C, alternate view

YOGA REST/CORPSE POSE

(Shavasana)

Begin in Sitting Mountain.

LOWER BODY: Shift your buttocks and upper body back to sit with your spine resting against the back of the chair. Choose to either:

A. Keep your legs and feet in Sitting Mountain;

B. Position a block or blocks under your feet at a lower height; with your knees bent, extend your legs out as far as is comfortable, resting the soles of your feet on the block(s); or

C. Position a bolster or stack of blocks at a higher height; straighten your legs and bring your heels to rest on the bolster or blocks, allowing your feet to splay out.

UPPER BODY: With your torso resting comfortably against the back of the chair, choose to either:

A. Keep your hands in Sitting Mountain, palms resting down on the thighs;

B. Place your hands in your lap, palms up, with one hand resting in the palm of the other hand in Dhyana Mudra; or

C. Place a prop or props behind your back, under your arms, and/or around your neck; place the backs of your hands on your thighs, palms facing up.

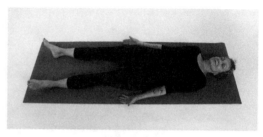

Yoga Rest/Corpse Pose, on the mat

BENEFITS: PHYSICAL
- Lowers blood pressure
- Calms nervous system
- Relaxes the body
- Supports digestive and immune systems
- Reduces fatigue

BENEFITS: MENTAL
- Calms and relaxes the mind
- Reduces stress and fatigue

EYE FOCUS
- Downward
- Eyes closed or soft

COUNTERPOSE
- Child's Pose

Putting it all together: We offer "Yoga Rest Pose" as an alternative English translation of *Shavasana* to help access a state of conscious repose. Come into this most versatile posture for relaxation at the end of a yoga session or for practicing breathing (chapter 8) or meditation (chapter 11). If you have chosen option C, make sure you've used enough props so that you can comfortably rest your whole body. Keep your gaze soft, casting your eyes downward or closing them. Come out of the pose slowly and return to Sitting Mountain.

Tips: Use props when available to support your body for maximum comfort. We recommend using a bolster, blocks, or a footstool under your feet; cushions or a rolled-up yoga mat behind your back; cushions under your elbows or arms; a rolled-up blanket around your neck, with the ends secured under your armpits; blankets over your body to retain warmth while at rest. You may discover other props that work better for you; see page 215 for more on props and assists. Bring your hands into any comfortable position, resting them on your thighs with your palms facing down (Chin Mudra), your palms facing up (Jnana Mudra), or any position of your choice; see pages 206–9 for other traditional mudra options.

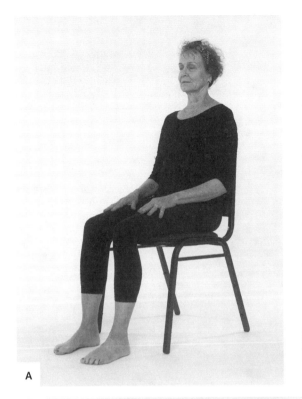

A

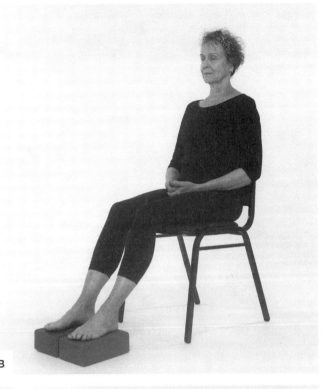

B

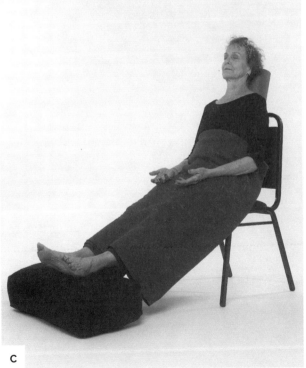

C

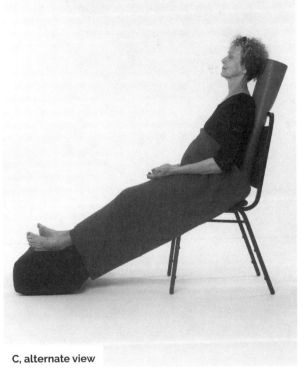

C, alternate view

10

Meditation, Relaxation, Mindfulness

Wisdom comes with the ability to be still. Just look and just listen.
No more is needed. . . . Let stillness direct your words and actions.

—ECKHART TOLLE, *The Power of Now*

IN THIS CHAPTER, we offer tips on how to experience and teach meditation and Shavasana (the traditional mat Yoga Rest Pose) on a chair safely and joyfully. Plus, we provide examples of several meditation styles we enjoy bringing to the chair.

Meditation has a long history, appearing in many traditions—religious, mystic, and mainstream—in both Eastern and Western cultures. In yoga, it is generally acknowledged that the practice of meditation brings clarity to the mind and fosters healing in the body. Today, many research studies have shown that practicing meditation positively supports health and wellness. By training our mindfulness "muscle," meditation helps bring our awareness into the present, helps reduce our tendency to ruminate on the past or obsess about the future, helps shift reactionary judgments, and encourages acceptance of our own thoughts and of "what is." And these practices are accessible to everyone at any moment!

In our chair-yoga approach, meditation can be practiced in conjunction with a focus on breath and/or movement, and it can be used as a stand-alone technique. It is a key aspect of any yoga practice: when the body moves and breathes, the heart beats faster and energy is created through the activation of the sympathetic nervous system—the fight-or-flight mode—while meditating after movement allows the body to relax and access the parasympathetic "rest-and-digest" aspect of the nervous system. By sitting up on our chairs to meditate, we not only "unload" and balance the spine, but we also do the same with the nervous system—the body-mind learns how to regulate and reduce stress in a healthy way.

While many images of meditation show participants seated cross-legged on the ground or on a cushion, and Shavasana is most often performed lying on the back, all meditation and relaxation practices can be done seated on a chair. Attention to postural alignment is essential when meditating on a chair to keep the spine safe and allow the breath, lungs, and diaphragm to move freely. To begin, come into a variation of Sitting Mountain that allows comfort and ease as well as the spine to remain lengthened. For example, some people like to sit farther back on the chair seat with a cushion behind to keep the spine upright. Others may put blocks or books under their feet or, when sitting on an armchair or wheelchair, tuck cushions underneath their elbows on one or both sides of the body. As body temperature often lowers when coming into stillness, it's nice to have a blanket or extra layers of clothing on hand. See Yoga Rest Pose on pages 180–81 for some options for relaxing or meditating on a chair.

Like other yoga techniques, meditation can serve as a form of self-care, with proven benefits in stress reduction. As with movement and breath, first ask yourself, "What is my intention? What am I trying to achieve?" Some common goals of meditation are bringing calmness and relaxation to the body and/or mind, developing present-moment awareness, finding inspiration, enhancing well-being, and connecting more deeply with oneself and others.

Once you know your intention, consider the style of meditation—and there are many to choose from. Meditation allows us to "tune in" to our inner selves (thoughts, feelings, emotions), and most meditation practices invite the body to be still as a prelude to quieting the mind. Can you or would you like to begin in stillness, or is pausing in this manner too challenging? To access inner stillness, consider these ideas, options, and tips:

- Start with a short meditation—even just sitting quietly for one minute or taking three breaths counts!—and build up slowly according to ability and interest.

- Close your eyes or keep them open with a softly focused downward gaze.

- Count your breaths. For example, inhale for a count of one and exhale for a count of two—to keep your awareness focused on your breath. Most meditation practices involve following the movement of the breath in and out as an easily accessible way to be mindful. When the mind wanders or is distracted, as inevitably happens, just gently bring your attention back to your breath.

- Try a guided meditation. Guided meditations often include visualizations, which provide a focus for the mind and an anchor for remaining in the present moment. Listening to the sound of someone else's voice (or even your own) can ease the mind and calm the heart. Feel free to record the meditation scripts in this book and modify them as you wish.

- Do a moving meditation. Flowing yoga styles such as vinyasa or Kripalu and relaxing body-mind practices such as qigong can be adapted to the chair to bring the body-mind into the present moment through movement, encouraging the nervous system to shift from energetic to relaxation mode. See the walking meditation on page 194 to discover how to walk while sitting up on a chair!

- Use hand gestures (mudras). Subtle movements like these are often effective in aiding concentration and helping the body-mind to access the benefits of meditation. (See page 206 in chapter 12 for more on mudras.)

- Incorporate visualizations, affirmations, or other yoga techniques such as chanting or mantras (see chapters 6 and 12). These techniques can help bring you into the present moment, giving you access to the wonderful benefits of mindfulness. As mentioned above, visualizations are often used in guided meditations, or feel free to come up with your own mental images.

- To help with motivation and for those new to meditation, consider signing up for a meditation class, using a meditation app, or finding a friend to "train" with—like an exercise buddy—to support each other as you learn.

THREE-MINUTE CHAIR YOGA FOR RELAXATION

When life is busy, there never seems to be enough time to relax, which is so necessary for managing stress and maintaining good health and wellness. How can we find time to recharge our batteries—get some actual "breathing space"—on a daily basis? You don't need to invest a lot of time to create space for relaxing your body-mind. Take a break from whatever you're doing—at home, work, school, on the road, wherever you are—and do this short practice. Research shows that it takes a minimum of three minutes for the body-mind to enter a state of relaxation,[13] so give it a try. It'll do you a world of good.

Come into Sitting Mountain on your chair, focusing on the cues that bring you into postural alignment. Silently or aloud set an intention, such as "Time for a pause to reset." Place (or imagine) one hand on your chest and one on your belly and take three slow breaths, noticing your breath flowing in and out of the body and the movement of your body as it breathes.

From Sitting Mountain, warm up any stiff joints—your choice. Get your ankles moving by coming up onto the ball of one foot and circling your ankle a few times. Or lift your foot off the ground to rotate it. Repeat on the other side. Now rotate your shoulders and wrists. Loosen your knees by sliding each leg forward and back, one at a time, or by lifting your thigh (using your hands underneath to assist if you'd like) and swinging your leg forward and back. Turn your head from side to side to release your neck, then tilt one ear down to your shoulder and back up again, and then do the same on the other side.

Now, sit all the way back on your chair while keeping the spine lengthened. With your eyes closed or with a soft downward gaze, breathe slowly and deeply into the abdomen for a few breaths, visualizing an image that is calming and relaxing, or repeating an affirmation to yourself, either silently or aloud, such as "I am resting. I am releasing. I am relaxing."

Slowly return to Sitting Mountain, then resume whatever you were doing, with gratitude for this brief gift of space.

Mindfulness on the Chair

Mindfulness as a practice has ancient roots, stemming in particular from Buddhist traditions, and it has become popular in many of today's societies as modern scientific research confirms its many wellness benefits, such as relieving stress and improving mental health.[14]

Mindfulness can be described as being in the present moment—being aware of one's thoughts, surroundings, and feelings in the here and now. Paying attention in the present moment allows you to respond with curiosity and without judgment rather than just react. At times, your mind may get carried away with ruminating on the past or anticipating the future, which can make you feel stressed, down, or anxious. If you have physical ailments, sometimes all you can seem to focus on is pain and discomfort. Being mindful—staying in the present moment—gives your mind a rest. It can take you out of yourself to help you cope better with painful situations and sensations.

In our experience, all meditation practices are mindful, while not all mindfulness practices have to be meditations! One of our favorite ways to explore present-moment experience is through an activity we do daily while seated: eating. Mindful eating involves focusing on one or more of your external senses (sight, sound, smell, taste, touch), such as noticing the shape and color of your food or chewing deliberately to examine the texture or to savor the flavors. By slowing down the eating process, you can enjoy your food more as well as improve digestion. In fact, any activity can be done mindfully just by bringing your attention to whatever task is at hand.

As you explore your own mindfulness practice or guide others as a teacher, remember these inspiring words written by Thich Nhat Hanh in *Peace Is Every Step*: "Peace is present right here and now, in ourselves and in everything we do and see. Every breath we take, every step we take, can be filled with peace, joy, and serenity. The question is whether or not we are in touch with it. We need only to be awake, alive in the present moment."

Applying the Yamas and Niyamas to Meditation

Meditation is personal to each one of us, and patience and dedication are important. Some can sit and meditate for over an hour or more, and others can barely sit for five minutes. Any length is fine—it depends on what is going on at the time for each individual. You can use visualizations, observe your breath coming in and going out, count each breath, recite a mantra, use a mudra or a *japamala* (meditation beads): whatever technique will lead you to settle, focus, and find contentment.

In meditation, we can apply the yamas (social restraints) and niyamas (personal observances) to our personal practice. When we do, we can come to increased awareness and better understanding.

AHIMSA: You can practice ahimsa (nonviolence) when you meditate by finding a comfortable place and way to sit that suits (and isn't harmful to) your body. If you find you're starting to berate yourself for not being able to meditate for as long as someone else, pause. Remind yourself to be kind and that it's just fine to sit for as long as you wish—whatever works from day to day. If your mind wanders (which it will), gently bring your attention back to your breath or the focus of the meditation, without self-judgment or self-criticism.

SATYA: You also practice satya (truthfulness) when you ask yourself, "Is this the correct time, place, and style of meditation for me?" If we start to meditate but the conditions are not right, then it's okay not to meditate. When we are truthful with ourselves, we are better able to access the joy and relaxation that meditation can bring.

ASTEYA: To practice asteya (nonstealing), we do not spend precious meditation time worrying about how someone else meditates or for how long. We do what is right for us on a day-to-day basis.

BRAHMACHARYA: Some suggest that meditation should be done for twenty minutes, an hour, or even a day, which may not be available to us. To practice brahmacharya (moderation), we remember that five minutes of meditation is always more beneficial than no minutes. Even one minute will do!

APARIGRAHA: With aparigraha (nonpossessiveness), you don't get attached to a particular outcome of your practice. There's no such thing as a "bad" meditation or a "good" meditation. Nor do you get attached to one form of meditating; there are many ways to meditate. It's up to you to find the way that works for you.

SAUCHA: Practicing saucha (purity) cultivates steadiness of mind during your meditation time, bringing your attention back to your breath or intention whenever your mind wanders.

SANTOSHA: Santosha (contentment) can come in choosing a meditation practice and being at peace with that choice, as you sit in the silence of your breath or whatever technique you've selected.

TAPAS: Tapas (self-discipline) is the willpower to commit to and show up for your meditation practice no matter what. To sit and watch your breath and be willing to finish your meditation when it feels right without judging yourself (*ahimsa*).

SVADHYAYA: Svadhyaya (self-education) comes into play when you do research and ask questions of others about meditation to help you decide what is best for you. Not for someone else—for you! Svadhyaya also allows you to notice the effects of your practice—as it is happening in real time.

ISHVARA PRANIDHANA: In finding or creating the time for a regular practice, we begin to slowly become aware of the ego's hold on us. Meditation creates a solid ground so that we may come, in time, to realize a divine life, ishvara pranidhana—one of peace and quietude as we begin to surrender our wants, needs, and desires to a higher power, whoever or whatever that may be. In time, our ego will surrender to our practice, and we will find happiness.

Below we describe five different meditation techniques on the chair, offering either step-by-step instructions or a full script. (See also pages 202–3 for a meditation script using the chakras as a theme.) As mentioned above, feel free to modify the scripts based on your own (or your students') preferences, and record them if you wish to listen to the voice of a teacher, another person, or yourself to help engage Patanjali's fifth limb of yoga, pratyahara (withdrawal of the senses), and experience true inner exploration.

Meditation and mindfulness practices that cultivate nonjudgmental awareness and enable true relaxation of the body-mind are challenging! A longtime student of our chair-yoga approach put it so succinctly: "Before I started to do yoga, the concept of stillness was completely foreign to me. Studying Patanjali's sutra on nurturing friendliness, compassion, delight, and disregard (1:33) led me to discover ways of accessing 'serenity of mind,' which has helped me handle the stresses of life. Over time, I've come to embrace meditative practices, especially moving meditations. Even breathing becomes a moving meditation when I focus on the diaphragm—that wonderful muscle that moves up and down like a parachute!" Be patient with and kind to yourself as you explore what works best. It is worth making and taking the time and space to discover which practices work best for you and, if you teach, for your students.

Breath Exploration

Our breath is amazing. We have the ability to bring conscious attention to it, yet it continues to flow regardless of whether we are conscious of it or not. We also have the power to energize or calm the body-mind just by altering our breath ourselves. The ancient yogis recognized this ability and power, and now modern science has shown that working intentionally with your breath can support good health and wellness. To train your ability and harness the power of your breath, get to know your own breath! This meditation on mindfulness of the breath provides one way to explore by guiding you to focus on different aspects of your breath, such as its location, speed, quality, and length. If the mind drifts or is distracted during the meditation, just bring it back to your natural breath or one aspect of your breath, being mindful to simply observe your breath with curiosity and without judgment.

BREATH EXPLORATION
Step-by-Step Instructions

Sit comfortably in Sitting Mountain or Yoga Rest Pose, settling yourself into a position where you can remain still. Close your eyes or gaze downward, letting your eyes focus softly. Now bring your attention to your breath, to the natural flow of your inbreath and outbreath. If you wish, place one hand on your chest and one on your abdomen, which will help you access your breath more easily.

First, notice where you feel your breath in your body. Is it in your nostrils, chest, rib cage, abdomen? Inhale and exhale naturally for one or more rounds while observing the location of your breath. Next, notice the speed and rhythm of your breath. Is it fast, slow, even, uneven? Inhale and exhale naturally for one or more rounds while observing the tempo of your breath.

Now, notice the quality of your breath. Is it smooth, choppy, shallow, deep? Inhale and exhale naturally for one or more rounds while observing the quality of your breath.

Finally, notice the length of your breath. Are the inhale and exhale the same length or is one longer than the other? Inhale and exhale naturally for one or more rounds while observing the length of the inhale and the exhale.

Return to noticing your breath flowing into and out of your nostrils for a few rounds before coming slowly back to an external awareness. Or continue your exploration by altering your breath using one of the techniques in chapter 8 or any other breathing technique of your choice.

Body Scan

Body scans are a type of formal mindful meditation. The idea is to concentrate on one part of your body at a time, paying attention with curiosity to how that body part feels, without trying to change anything. Move mentally through your body, lingering on each body part as long as you like. By noticing sensations in this structured fashion, we can get to know our body and learn to be with our feelings and emotions—including challenging ones such as pain, anger, and fear—in calmer and more composed ways. Body scans can help with relaxation as well as provide relief from stress, anxiety, or physical challenges; they can also be used to generate more energy in the body-mind. The instructions below offer a guide to creating a body scan that you can do on your own or, if you teach, with your students.

BODY SCAN
Step-by-Step Instructions

Sit comfortably in Sitting Mountain or Yoga Rest Pose, settling yourself into a position where you can remain still. Close your eyes or gaze downward, letting your eyes focus softly. Now bring your attention to your breath, to the natural flow of your inbreath and outbreath. Start either at the top of your head or the tips of your toes and work down or up from there.

Place your awareness on that first body part. Notice any sensations, such as tingling, pulsing, warmth, coolness. Inhale and focus your breath on this body part. Then exhale any tension before moving your awareness to the next body part.

Take as much or as little time as you wish by adding or skipping body parts and/or increasing the number of breaths focused on each body part. Continue to explore the sensations as they arise.

Repeat until you have reached the opposite end of your body. Return to your natural breath for a few rounds before coming back to an external awareness.

Loving-Kindness Meditation (*Metta*)

A type of guided visualization with origins in Buddhist traditions, loving-kindness meditation encourages an open and giving heart. Its Sanskrit name, *metta*, translates as "loving-kindness," and the idea is to send wishes of happiness and peace to others as well as ourselves. It can include dedicating the practice to a particular person, a group of people, or all of humankind and beyond through the repetition of a series of affirmations or phrases. (See chapter 11 for more on affirmations.) This meditation is said to improve concentration, foster connection, and support feelings of safety through kindness and positivity (*ahimsa*). The script below focuses on the theme of compassion; feel free to adapt the theme or the affirmations (using more or fewer) to suit yourself or, if you teach, your students.

LOVING-KINDNESS MEDITATION

Script[15]

Sit comfortably in Sitting Mountain or Yoga Rest Pose, settling yourself into a position where you can remain still. Close your eyes or gaze downward, letting your eyes focus softly. Now bring your attention to your breath, to the natural flow of your inbreath—your inhale—and your outbreath—your exhale. The breath is a source of life, all life, and it connects us to a sense of compassion and kindness for ourselves and others. Now focus on these words, repeating the following phrases silently to yourself, in your mind:

> *May I be happy and peaceful.*
>
> *May I be nourished and well.*
>
> *May I look after myself with contentment and joy.*
>
> *May I possess the patience, courage, steadfastness, and wisdom to meet the challenges of my life.*

Finally, send this loving-kindness to yourself, bathing yourself in the light of compassion and acceptance.

Now think of someone you love or respect and bring them into your awareness. Say these phrases to yourself:

> *May this person that I love/respect be happy and peaceful.*
>
> *May they be nourished and well.*
>
> *May they look after themselves with contentment and joy.*
>
> *May they possess the patience, courage, steadfastness, and wisdom to meet the challenges of their life.*

Finally, send loving-kindness to this person, bathing them in the light of compassion and understanding.

Now bring to mind someone you've seen, perhaps in your neighborhood or at work, but whom you don't know well. Whether you're aware of it or not, this person, like you, also has challenges, experiencing both joy and pain. Repeat these phrases to yourself:

> *May this person be happy and peaceful.*
>
> *May they be nourished and well.*
>
> *May they look after themselves with contentment and joy.*
>
> *May they possess the patience, courage, steadfastness,*
>   *and wisdom to meet the challenges of their life.*

Finally, send loving-kindness to this person, bathing them in the light of compassion and consideration.

Now let's extend our awareness to all beings, all life. Realize that all life has its challenges, its pain, and its joy. Say these phrases to yourself:

> *May all beings be happy and peaceful.*
>
> *May they be nourished and well.*
>
> *May they look after themselves with contentment and joy.*
>
> *May they possess the patience, courage, steadfastness,*
>   *and wisdom to meet the challenges of existence.*

Finally, send loving-kindness to all beings, bathing all life in the light of compassion, acceptance, understanding, and consideration.

Now bring this awareness back to yourself. Sitting where you are in your space. Part of all of life. Think again of your challenges and your joys, repeating these words to yourself:

> *May I be happy and peaceful.*
>
> *May I be nourished and well.*
>
> *May I look after myself with contentment and joy.*
>
> *May I possess the patience, courage, steadfastness,*
>   *and wisdom to meet the challenges of my life.*

Finally, send this loving-kindness to yourself, bathing yourself in the light of compassion and loving-kindness.

Now return to focus on your natural breath, your life energy, breathing in and breathing out. Trust that being more with your breath and the light of compassion will help you through life's challenges, reducing tension, giving you energy, connecting you to more than yourself. When you're ready, come back slowly to awareness of the space around you in whatever way is most comfortable, ready to resume your day.

Yoga Nidra

Yoga Nidra, which translates as "yogic sleep," is a guided meditation that brings about a state of consciousness somewhere between sleeping and waking. It leads you through a series of verbal instructions that gradually draws the attention inward and away from the external senses (*pratyahara*) into a state of complete relaxation. While a body scan often takes a linear journey through the body with a focus on sensation awareness, Yoga Nidra guides conscious awareness around the body in a rotating sequence, progressing from part to part; other elements such as visualization, intention, and a comparison of opposites (*pratipaksha bhavana*) may be incorporated. This type of meditation is said to develop self-awareness, increase focus, and foster deep body-mind relaxation. Usually practiced lying down in a comfortable position, you can also practice Yoga Nidra on a chair. The script below provides a simple example; feel free to record it and follow your own voice through the practice, choosing a chair and place of your liking. There are many forms of Yoga Nidra, varying from five minutes to an hour in length, which can be accessed in meditation classes or online. We encourage you to explore to find ones that work for you and, if you teach, your students.

YOGA NIDRA

Script[16]

Sit comfortably in Sitting Mountain or Yoga Rest Pose. Add anything you need—cushions, blankets, props—to feel more at ease, so your body can rest fully on the chair. Take time to arrange yourself so that you can relax and let the weight of your body drop down onto the chair seat and your feet sink down onto the ground. Be as comfortable as possible, allowing your body to be fully supported underneath you.

Now allow yourself to follow the gentle flow of your breath in and out. With each exhalation, feel yourself letting go into what is supporting you; let the chair and the earth hold you. Feel the contact points where your body meets the chair and the ground. Tune in to those contact points: the touch at the back of your body, on the seat of the chair, on the ground below your feet. With each exhalation, allow those contact points to melt into the earth: your spine and the back of the chair; your buttocks and the chair seat; your feet and the ground; your whole body and the legs or wheels of the chair.

Start to feel all the contact points where your body and its support meet, all at the same time. You can imagine that the contact points are merging with the chair and the ground, sinking with each exhalation. Or you can imagine that there are weighted strings coming from those contact points so that each time you exhale, they are lovingly pulling you to the core of the earth. With each inhalation, feel that you are free and light: the front of your body is free, your belly and ribs are expanding to welcome the fullness of the inhalation, the crown of your head is lifting softly toward the sky. Imagine you are as light as a feather, almost as if you are floating away.

Spend a few minutes gently playing with the opposite sensations of lightness with the inhalation and the sense of grounding connection to the core of the earth with the exhalation. If it feels comfortable and safe to do so, let your breath become long and deep.

As you feel your body settle, let go of any physical tension you can, and see if you are able to remain still for the rest of the practice. Of course, if you need to move, that's fine—make sure you feel safe and comfortable throughout.

Now bring your attention to the space between your eyebrows, the "Third Eye" center. All attention on the space between the eyebrows—just let your attention settle there. Imagine a bright light shining from this space. Now move your attention to the soft hollow of your throat. Again, visualize a bright light shining there. Now move your attention to your right shoulder, imagining a light there, then to your right elbow and your right wrist, again seeing bright lights in both those places. Then see bright lights on each of the tips of your thumb, index finger, middle finger, ring finger, and little finger of your right hand. Now trace all those little lights back, like constellations of stars, through your right wrist, elbow, shoulder, and back to the soft hollow of your throat.

Now move your attention to your left shoulder, imagining a light there, then to your left elbow and your left wrist, again seeing bright lights in both those places. Then see bright lights on each of the tips of your thumb, index finger, middle finger, ring finger, and little finger of your left hand. Now trace all those little lights back, like constellations of stars, through your wrist, elbow, shoulder, and back to the soft hollow of your throat.

Now move your attention to the center of your chest. See a bright light shining from the space behind the center of your chest, the breastbone. Light now moves to the right side of your chest, back to the center of your chest, and then over to the left side of your chest. And back to the center behind the breastbone.

Now move your attention down to your abdomen—a bright light at the navel. Then to the center of your pelvic floor, the base of your abdomen—bright shining light. Now move to your right hip, bright light at your right hip, then bright lights at your right knee, ankle, and toes, lighting one toe at a time. Trace that constellation of lights back from your right toes, ankle, knee, and hip to the center of your pelvic floor. Now move to your left hip, bright light at the left hip, then bright lights at your left knee, ankle, and toes, lighting one toe at a time. Trace that constellation of lights back from your left toes, ankle, knee, and hip to the center of your pelvic floor.

Now move your attention—bright lights—to your navel, the center of your chest, the hollow of your throat, and back to the space between your eyebrows. Continue to hold your attention at the space between your eyebrows now, allowing thoughts and images to drift by like clouds moving through the sky. All thoughts, all images, all emotions passing by like light clouds moving through the sky. Finally, bring your attention to your heart space, the space at the center of your rib cage, the center of your being. Rest your attention there, offering any gratitude you feel moved to offer, and offering any intentions that feel right to you. You can even be open to receiving any messages from your own deep intuition.

Gradually bring your attention back to your breath. Feel your body breathing and allow your breath to guide you back to your body. Feel your body sitting on the chair, feel the contact points between your body, the chair, and the ground once again. Feel your body resting on the chair and the expansion and relaxation of your ribs, chest, and belly as your breath flows in and out. Start to breathe a little deeper, taking each inhalation as a source of energy, bringing you back to your body in the here and now. Gently come back to the external senses: notice any smells, tastes, sounds. Bring your attention to the sense of touch and start to move and stretch in any way you wish. Finally, when you are ready, gently open your eyes and slowly come back to awareness and to the room, the space, the environment around you.

Seated Walking Meditation

The benefits of walking are widely documented, including improved fitness as well as preventing and managing a range of cardiovascular and other conditions. But not everyone is able to physically stand and walk. Even for those who can, it's not always convenient—for instance, when working or traveling. And while many meditation practices expect the body to remain still, not everyone is able to access a quiet and unmoving state. As an alternative, we recommend a seated walking meditation, which can be done on any chair, anywhere!

Walking meditation, whether seated or standing, involves structured walking movements and the use of mental images or descriptions for these movements. This practice can aid concentration, improve body awareness, and release energy and stress. As with asana practice, intentionally moving the body keeps the mind in the present moment, and a seated walking meditation can be an accessible prelude to sitting in stillness. Below we offer some steps as a guide—feel free to play with these suggestions and create your own seated walking meditation or, if you teach, one that inspires your students.

SEATED WALKING MEDITATION
Step-by-Step Instructions[17]

Come into Sitting Mountain, with the soles of your feet on the ground and your palms down on your thighs. Become aware of your breath as it flows in and out of your nostrils. Breathe naturally for a few rounds. Feel the touch of your palms on your legs and the soles of your feet on the ground.

If you wish, start your practice by bringing to mind this affirmation, or choose one of your own, repeating it aloud or silently to yourself: "Let my movements, breath, and thoughts harmonize with the world all around, like a surfer riding a wave."

Begin by raising one heel slowly off the ground (or lift your entire foot) and silently say, "Lifting." As you put your heel or foot slowly back down, say to yourself, "Placing." Keeping the soles of both feet flat on the ground, make a mental note, "Pausing." Repeat the movements and descriptions with your other heel or foot.

Now repeat the physical movements and mental descriptions with each hand, slowly raising the heel of each hand, or lift your whole hand, in turn.

Continue to "walk" with your feet and hands in any combination you wish—mix and match!—describing each movement in your mind. If available, inhale to align with one movement and exhale to align with the next, coordinating the movement with each breath. At the end of the practice, release and return to Sitting Mountain and awareness of your natural breath.

Tips: Keep the pace of your walk slow and steady, or begin at a faster rate and slow down as you progress.

When first practicing this meditation, start with a few rounds of one to three minutes, then build up gradually to ten to twenty minutes (as available).

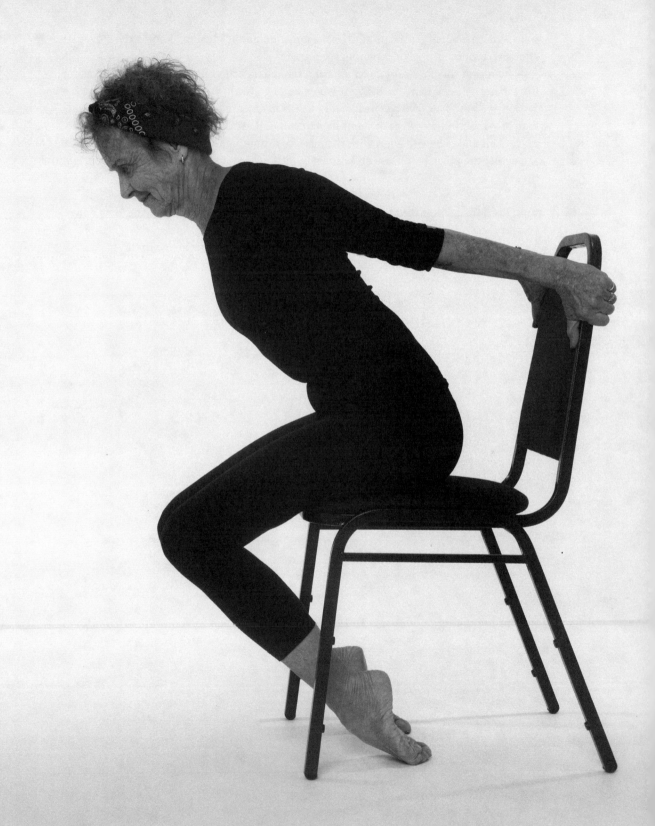

PART FOUR

Supplementals

11

More Joy on the Chair

Chakras, Chanting, Mantras, and Mudras

Yoga is the golden key that unlocks the door to peace, tranquility, and joy.

—B. K. S. IYENGAR

IT HAS BEEN SAID, "If you can't find joy in a pose, you're not doing yoga," which could easily be the tagline for our approach to chair yoga. This chapter focuses on just a few yoga techniques—incorporating the chakras, chanting and mantras, and mudras (gestures)—that add extra variety and joy to the experience and that can serve as powerful tools for promoting balance and wellness to body, mind, and spirit. In fact, in our experience, any technique or style of yoga can be adapted to the chair. In our own chair-yoga practice and teacher training, we include a wealth of other movements and body-mind activities adapted to the chair. In addition to the single-chair yoga explored in this book, we teach double-chair yoga, pair-chair (partner) yoga, and weighted chair yoga; dance moves, acupressure massage, reflexology, and qigong are wonderful additions to any chair-yoga class. We encourage you to explore our suggestions and, more importantly, bring your creativity and your sat nam—your own voice and personal identity—to the chair.

Chakras on the Chair

The word *chakra* translates from the Sanskrit as "wheel" or "circle." Yoga defines the chakras as centers of energy in the astral body: six of them are located along the spine, with the first, or "root," chakra at the base and the seventh chakra at the crown of the head. Each is associated with different qualities, such as a sound vibration, a color, and an element. We cannot see the

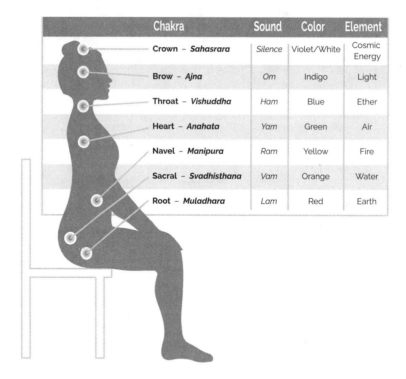

Chakra	Sound	Color	Element
Crown – *Sahasrara*	Silence	Violet/White	Cosmic Energy
Brow – *Ajna*	Om	Indigo	Light
Throat – *Vishuddha*	Ham	Blue	Ether
Heart – *Anahata*	Yam	Green	Air
Navel – *Manipura*	Ram	Yellow	Fire
Sacral – *Svadhisthana*	Vam	Orange	Water
Root – *Muladhara*	Lam	Red	Earth

chakras: they are subtle energy fields within the body. It is said that when a chakra is blocked, "dis-ease" can occur; working with the chakras through yoga can restore balance and wellness to body, mind, and spirit.

We can access and work with the chakras in a multitude of ways. For example, focusing on one or more of them as a theme for a meditation or for an entire class, or choosing one of the qualities, depending on the intention. Below are some chakra exercises, affirmations, and a meditation script that can be used by practitioners and teachers to balance and heal internal energies.

CHAKRA EXERCISES AND AFFIRMATIONS

First Chakra: *Muladhara*—Root Chakra—I Am

Security and survival. Finding your purpose in life. Growing roots and grounding.

"I open to receive the gift of life."

Sit near the front edge of your chair, placing your hands beside you on the seat of the chair. Lift your buttocks up and then gently down. Repeat six more times, pushing the press points in your feet onto the ground while visualizing the color red.

Second Chakra: *Svadhishthana*—Sacral Chakra—I Feel

Identity, creativity, and sexuality. Flowing with change.

"I am a unique manifestation of energy in physical form. I dance in harmony with the rhythm of that energy."

Make fists with your hands and place them on either your hip flexors or your groin area. Press in and breathe deeply for thirty seconds while visualizing the color orange.

Third Chakra: *Manipura*—Navel Chakra—I Do

The power center of the body. Finding our will, purpose, and action.

"I open to the fullness of my power. I have within me the power to create, sustain, and transform."

Place your hands on your knees. Lift your chest to open the front body and arch your upper back, bringing your shoulder blades toward each other, then drop your chin toward your chest and lift your upper back to gently curl and open your spine, alternating forward and backward. Do these movements six more times while visualizing the color yellow.

Fourth Chakra: *Anahata*—Heart Chakra—I Love

Love and compassion. Living in our hearts from our hearts.

"I open to the depth of love that dwells within me. I am love, I receive love, and I give love."

Open your arms out to your sides and back, palms facing forward. Raise your chest up and out. Bring your palms together in front of your heart, gently curling the spine. Repeat six more times while visualizing the color green.

Fifth Chakra: *Vishuddha*—Throat Chakra—I Speak

Center of expression. Communicating our hearts to the world.

"I open to the universal truth within me. I receive it. I share it."

Turn your head slowly side to side eight times, then up and down eight times, while visualizing the color blue.

Sixth Chakra: *Ajna*—Brow or Third-Eye Chakra—I See

The center of meditation, contemplation, visualization, affirmation, and intellect. Awakening our intuition.

"I open to the wisdom that dwells within me. I open to my guidance."

Sit up tall in Sitting Mountain, place your palms behind you on your chair seat with your fingers pointing away from you. Focus your eyes on the high seam and breathe deeply, then close your eyes and focus on the "Third Eye"—the space between your eyebrows. Continue for as long as you want while visualizing the color indigo.

Seventh Chakra: *Sahasrara*—Crown Chakra—I Understand

Governs universal consciousness, enlightenment, our connection with all that is. Connecting to a higher power.

"I am one with all."

Sit in Sitting Mountain with your spine against the chair back. Place the back of one hand in the palm of your other hand on your lap, palms facing up, thumbs and index fingers touching in Dhyana Mudra. Close your eyes and focus on your breath for a few minutes while visualizing the color violet.

Finish by focusing on a healing white light surrounding your body-mind.

Chakra Meditation

Below is a guided meditation script using the chakras as a theme. The visualizations bring attention to the seven areas of the body outlined above. To enhance this awareness, place a hand (or two) on each area, or imagine doing this, as the meditation progresses. Feel free to adapt the script if you wish—for instance, by either keeping the Sanskrit names for the chakras or taking out the word *chakra* entirely.

CHAKRA MEDITATION
Script

Sit comfortably on your chair, feet flat on the ground, palms gently placed down on your thighs. Close your eyes or have a soft downward gaze, bringing your awareness to the flow of your breath, relaxing your belly, calming your mind. Take a moment to notice your natural breath, the rhythm as it comes in on the inhale and as it goes out on the exhale, and let it flow freely.

Imagine that your breath, a beam of light, or a wheel of energy is entering from the crown of your head. Let this breath, this light, this wheel of energy travel down your body, parallel to your spine, all the way to your feet, connecting onto the ground below.

Now imagine this breath, this beam of light, this wheel slowing turning into an earthy russet or auburn color. Bring your attention to your feet on the ground and let the earth, stable and solid, support your root chakra: your feet, lower legs, knees, upper legs. Gradually feel the release of any stagnant or negative energy from your lower body, making space for a fresh flow of positive energy.

Now visualize your breath, the light, the wheel moving up to your buttocks and hips. Think of this area—the sacral chakra—as a flowing river. Imagine these flowing waters cleaning the energy to unblock any negativity or tension. Notice, if you will, the orange reflection of the sun in the waters, a sign of strength and vitality.

Next, bring your attention to your abdomen and lower back, imagining here at the navel chakra the yellow flames of a fire. Let your breath, the light, the wheel either fan or dampen the flames, whatever you need to nourish yourself, your willpower, your gut instinct, finding confidence and wisdom.

Now let's move up to your chest and midback where the heart chakra resides. Visualize pure, clean air entering the body here, settling in and then expanding into your heart. Perhaps it's clear, cold mountain air or the lush, rich atmosphere of a forest of green, filling you with courage and compassion.

Gently bring your attention to the area around your shoulders, neck, and upper back, imagining here space unfolding all around—the blue of sky or sea, or the openness of words or deeds. At the throat chakra, feel vibrations of positive energy, resonating truth and clarity.

Now come to focus on the space between the eyes—the brow chakra. Allow the vibrations here to resonate as a calm but powerful light, the color of indigo, that color between blue and violet, the deep purple of a starry night sky, reflecting insight and wisdom.

Now you come to the top of your head. Imagine here a violet glow or pure white energy as your breath, a beam of light, or a wheel spinning around at the crown chakra. Visualize and feel this pristine energy unblocking this final point, making way for all negative thoughts and energies to exit your body and for positive thoughts and energies to enter.

Let a rainbow of color now release from the crown, as your breath, the light, or the spinning wheel, flowing out and down to envelop your whole body with positive energy, healing, and peace.

Breathe naturally, allowing your body to fully relax with every breath, every inhale, and every exhale.

When you feel ready, gently awaken again—perhaps wiggling your toes and fingers or stroking your head with your fingers—and then stretch your body in whatever way feels good for you. In your own time, open your eyes and come back into Sitting Mountain.

Chanting and Mantras on the Chair

Babies in utero hear their mother's heartbeat and the sound of all the bodily fluids moving through both of their bodies. These sounds are the first sounds a baby hears, soothing the transition to the outer world from the comfort and security of a baby's first home. Chanting can take a child or adult back to that place of serenity and safety.

Chanting, like meditation, has an ancient history, with roots in every major religious tradition. It also has therapeutic qualities and can be wonderfully healing by replacing fear and anxiety with joy and a full heart. Often, those who cannot verbalize can instead communicate through music and sound. Research shows that music can decrease pain, calm fearful and anxious thoughts, improve mood and overall well-being, and facilitate present-moment awareness.[18]

Chants are composed of sounds or words, and in many yoga traditions, they are repeated in a songlike manner called a *mantra*, which translates from the Sanskrit as an "instrument of thought." Mantras composed of a one-syllable sound are called *bija* (seed) mantras. It is said that mantras, and seed mantras in particular, can create strong vibrations that resonate in body, mind, and spirit.

You can use a mantra anytime—by speaking it aloud or saying it silently to yourself. In our approach to chair yoga, teachers may introduce mantras at the beginning and/or end of a practice, or they can be used throughout as a theme that integrates a session. They are often used in meditation, repeated to aid concentration and foster stillness of the mind. Here are a few examples of mantras that we enjoy using on the chair:

- **OM** is a well-known seed mantra, considered the most sacred mantra in certain traditions. It consists of three sounds—*A-U-M*—and is associated with three main characteristics of creation, preservation, and liberation. It is sometimes referred to as "the sound of the universe," acknowledging our connection with all things as well as the entire cosmos.

  » *Practice tip:* Chant OM three times at the beginning and end of any session to bring the sound connection full circle.

- **CHAKRA SOUNDS** can also serve as seed mantras, chanting the sound of each chakra as the attention rests on its related section of the body (see illustration on page 200).

  » *Practice tip:* Incorporate the chanting of chakra sounds into the exercises or meditations above (pages 200–203) to enhance the benefits of focused awareness on each body area.

- **NAMASTE** is a noncontact respectful form of addressing another person, which translates as "I honor the light within you that resides within me."

  » *Practice tip:* When practicing with or teaching others, speak or chant *namaste* at the end of the session.

- **SHANTI** is simple yet profound in its meaning: "peace."

  » *Practice tip:* Chant *shanti* three times at the end of the session.

- **SAT NAM** means our "true self," our own authentic voice and identity (see page 28 for further details on sat nam, a key philosophical principle of our approach to chair yoga).

  » *Practice tip:* Come into Sitting Mountain and chant *sat nam* to yourself silently or aloud as many times as you wish, or chant it in the same way as *namaste* or *shanti*.

- **HAMSA** means "I am that." Sometimes expressed with the syllables inverted as *soham*, this mantra is a powerful one and a favorite of ours in our chair-yoga practice.

  » *Practice tip:* Come into Sitting Mountain and observe your breath flow in and out. Become aware of your breath repeating *ham-sa, ham-sa*. Focus on the syllables as they rise and subside: *ham* is the perfect "I"—the self—and *sa* is the universal energy—a higher power. "I am that."

  The *hamsa* mantra allows us to have a direct experience of the self. It can be practiced easily and effortlessly by anyone. There are mantras repeated with the tongue and those spoken while touching the beads of a japamala (meditation beads). *Hamsa* is different. Translated as "I am that, that I am, I AM," it emanates naturally from within, flowing seamlessly with any breathing technique: As the breath comes in, it makes the sound *ham*, and when it goes out, it makes the sound *sa*. For this reason, it can also be called "my own mantra" or the "mantra of the self."

While yoga chants and mantras are most often written and voiced in the language of Sanskrit, we can also use our own everyday language in a similar manner using affirmations. Affirmations are declarations that something is true, and we can use them as a way to state something that we wish to be or to accomplish. The Lakshmi Voelker Method's Sitting Mountain affirmation—"I am the mountain. I am stable. I am solid. I am secure. I am balanced" (page 41)—provides an embodied statement that supports good postural alignment. Repeating the words when we do this asana helps the body and the mind remember and assist each other, increasing our chances of gaining the benefits of the pose.

We encourage you to explore for yourself (and, if you teach, with your students) the option of chanting or not, voicing aloud or silently, honoring each individual's body-mind on that day. Feel free to come up with your own positive affirmations in the language of your choice, starting with the word *I*—this can be very empowering. Chanting opens the heart of the chanter to a connection with divine energy. To bring chanting to those in your chair-asana class is like bringing nectar to a hummingbird or pollen to a bee.

Mudras on the Chair

Mudra translates from the Sanskrit as "seal" or "sign." It is a symbolic or ritual gesture made with the hands, face, or body. Another meaning stems from its two root words: *mud* meaning "happiness" and *ra* meaning "to give." So a mudra may also be seen as a gesture that gives happiness—a physical expression of joy within. In our approach to chair yoga, we use hand mudras to build strength and bone mass by engaging the muscles of the hands and arms; maintain or improve flexibility in the fingers; cultivate attention and focus during any part of a yoga practice—breathing, movement, or meditation; and enhance our experience of doing yoga on a chair.

There are many hand mudras in yoga and all of them can be easily adapted for a chair-yoga practice. To modify them, you can simply visualize doing the full mudra or make the gesture with one hand only.

In this section, we outline a few of our favorites. See also chapter 8 for explanations of two mudras traditionally done with specific breathing techniques: Vishnu Mudra for Alternate Nostril Breathing (page 66) and Shanmukhi Mudra for Humming Bee Breath (page 69).

ADI MUDRA

Adi Mudra means "first seal." It is the first gesture a baby makes and is known as a gesture of stillness. Adi mudra has a soothing effect on the nervous system.

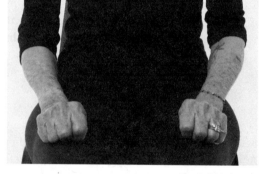

Adi Mudra

Instructions: Make fists by folding your thumbs into your palms and curling your four fingers over them. Place your fists on top of your thighs, palms down.

Practice: This gesture is said to provide grounding and stability, and it quiets the body-mind to support relaxation and calm. Bringing our hands into Adi Mudra, the hands' primal position inside the womb, can create serenity and tranquility, connecting us with creation and oneness with ourselves and the universe—we are all born with yoga in our DNA!

Selected poses: Sitting Mountain, Yoga Rest Pose

ANJALI MUDRA

Anjali Mudra means "divine offering" or "prayer of the heart." It is a gesture used in prayer, and it also serves as a greeting.

Instructions: Bring your palms together in front of your chest, either fully touching each other or with a small space in between your palms, and extend your fingers upward. The hands can be held away from your body or with the knuckles of your thumbs placed onto your sternum—at the heart center.

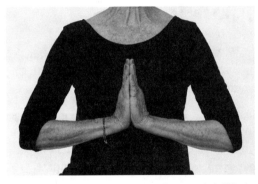

Anjali Mudra

Practice: This gesture is said to symbolize the unity of matter and spirit and help connect with the Divine in ourselves and in all beings. Asking with outstretched hands, palms together in front of the heart in Anjali Mudra, can represent the steadfast belief that whatever we are asking for will come to us in due time.

Selected poses: Sitting Mountain, Revolved Lunge, Squat Pose

CHIN MUDRA

Chin Mudra is known as a gesture of consciousness, often used in conjunction with Jnana Mudra, and helps improve inner awareness.

Instructions: Place your thumb and index finger together to make a circle, with the other three fingers lengthened out. Rest your hands on your thighs, palms facing down.

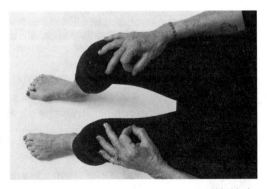

Chin Mudra

Practice: This gesture is said to support conscious awareness and connection to our higher self, with the downward-facing palms drawing energy from the earth below and the closed circle of the two fingers representing the union of body, mind, and spirit. In our chair-yoga practice, we often use this mudra to invite calmness or grounding to the body-mind.

Selected poses: Sitting Mountain, Victory Pose, Yoga Rest Pose

JNANA MUDRA

Jnana Mudra is known as a gesture of knowledge or wisdom, often used in conjunction with Chin Mudra.

Instructions: Place your thumb and index finger together to make a circle, with the other three fingers lengthened out. Place the backs of your hands on your thighs, palms facing up.

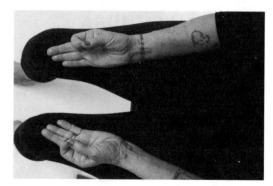

Jnana Mudra

Practice: This gesture is said to support clear understanding, tapping into one's intuition, with the upward-facing palms drawing divine energy from above and the closed circle of the two fingers representing unity of body, mind, and spirit. In our chair-yoga practice, we often use this mudra to invite energy into the body-mind.

Selected poses: Sitting Mountain, Extended One-Leg Pose, Victory Pose

DHYANA MUDRA

Dhyana Mudra is known as a gesture of reflection and meditation that has the ability to enable the mind to go deep into meditation.

Instructions: Place the back of one hand into the palm of the other on your lap, letting them come into the shape of a cup or bowl. Bring the outsides of your little fingers close to the lower abdomen and allow the tips of the thumbs to touch.

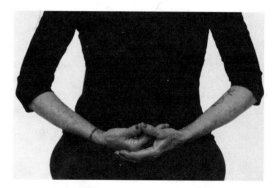

Dhyana Mudra

Practice: Sharing its name with Patanjali's seventh limb of yoga, this gesture is said to help access the benefits of meditation. According to some yoga traditions, placing the right hand on the left hand supports feminine energy associated with the moon and coolness, while placing the left hand on the right hand represents masculine energy associated with the sun and warmth.

Selected poses: Sitting Mountain, Tree Pose, Yoga Rest Pose

HAKINI MUDRA

Hakini Mudra means "power seal." It is known as a gesture of the brow (the "Third Eye") or forehead that helps control the mind and channel the flow of life-force energy.

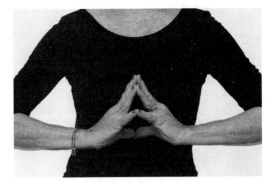
Hakini Mudra

Instructions: Bring the tips of your thumbs and all your fingers together in front of your solar plexus (upper abdomen). Open your palms and fingers, keeping your fingertips touching, into a rounded or tent shape.

Practice: This gesture is said to balance the left and right hemispheres of the brain, harmonizing and integrating all the body's systems, and to foster access to inner wisdom. Holding our hands in Hakini Mudra can encourage the assimilation all parts of the body-mind into an experience of wholeness and unity.

Selected poses: Sitting Mountain, Squat Pose, Tree Pose

PADMA MUDRA

Padma Mudra means "lotus seal." It is known as a gesture of the heart.

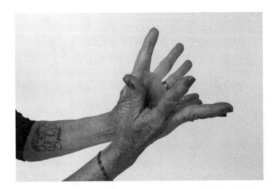
Padma Mudra

Instructions: Place the heels of your hands together. Bring your thumbs to touch each other, and your little fingers come together as well. Extend your fingers up and out into the shape of a flower, creating lotus petals by spreading your fingers wide.

Practice: This gesture may be associated with anahata chakra, the heart chakra, and is said to open the heart to compassion, empathy, sensitivity, and light. You are the jewel in the heart of the lotus!

Selected poses: Warrior I, High Lunge Pose

12

Safety on the Chair

Certainly you will have doubts. There will be questioning, and
faith will return again. This is how faith is established.

—SRI SARADA DEVI

MANY WONDERFUL RESOURCES exist on how yoga can help myriad conditions and
injuries, and it falls outside the scope of this book to cover them all. Instead, we explain how
awareness of a few basic precautions and levels of flexibility will allow teachers and students
to practice our approach to chair yoga safely in most circumstances. In addition, we provide
tips on how to practice and teach safely on any chair, how to set up a safe and welcoming space
for teaching and practicing, and how to safely use props and other "assists."

Precautions

In our chair-yoga approach, we speak about precautions rather than use the medical term
contraindications. The word *contraindication* suggests "cannot," and there is not one pose that
cannot be adapted and taught on the chair using levels of flexibility. When we are empowered
to find our own level while practicing chair yoga, we learn to listen to our bodies, tapping into
our inner resources, understanding, and wisdom about what works best for us—we are each
an expert on our own selves. Further, with knowledge of a few simple precautions, we can
focus instead on the benefits we gain from each yoga technique. For example, someone who
experiences migraines or tension headaches may choose to lift and fully lengthen their leg in
Extended One-Leg Pose (option C on page 111) as their lower-body level of flexibility. Yet this
same person may want to select a more basic level in Spinal Twist (options A or B on page 157)
to avoid neck strain, honoring the body-mind and still gaining benefits from the pose.

The main precautions for each pose in this book are included in chapter 9. For details about postural safety, please refer to chapter 6 on our principles of alignment.

While applying our levels of flexibility ensures a safe chair-yoga practice, there are specific points to be aware of as general precautions and for specific conditions:

- Avoid dropping your head back to keep the arteries and nerves in your neck safe. (See page 47 for more on neck safety and focusing the eyes.)

- Keep your shoulder joints safe by properly raising and lowering your arms (see page 48).

- Before coming into a twist, sit up tall in Sitting Mountain and lengthen your spine to protect your lower back. If you have osteoporosis, bone loss, or a spinal disc condition, be sure to lengthen your torso and hinge from your hips when forward folding and avoid deep rounding of your spine. (See page 50 for more details on spinal safety.)

- To avoid impingement in the hips, choose an alternative leg position as needed, according to levels of flexibility, as outlined on page 52.

- When focusing the eyes (*drishti*), you can always choose to keep your eyes open, half-open in a softened gaze, or closed.

- If you have high blood pressure that is not well controlled, keep your head above your heart when doing forward folds in case of lightheadedness, dizziness, or headaches to avoid risk of stroke. Avoid breath retention or fast movements. When raising your arms above your head, keep your neck in line with your spine and your head level, looking forward with your eyes, not up. Arms should also not remain above your head in a hold.

- For any issues with breathing, please refer to chapter 8.

- If you are deaf or have hearing challenges, sit toward the front when attending chair-yoga classes. Ask the teacher to provide clear visual cues and demonstrations of all yoga techniques and to avoid using background music while instructing so that anyone with hearing loss can hear the teacher's voice.

- If you have sight challenges, ask your teacher to provide clear and accurate verbal instructions.

- In case of allergies or asthma, ask your teacher to avoid the use of scents or essential oils.

- If you are pregnant, avoid variations of poses where your belly presses into your thighs. Also avoid twisting your abdomen.

- For any condition or injury, physical or mental, be sure to check with your doctor or health-care professional beforehand to make sure it is safe to practice chair yoga or any form of exercise.

About Chairs

We are often asked what's the best chair to use. In the Lakshmi Voelker Method, the chair becomes an extension of your body: your back is the back of the chair; your buttocks are the seat of the chair; the front chair legs are your two legs; and the back chair legs are your two sit bones. While our chair-yoga method can be adapted for use on any chair, it is important that the chair be stable and sturdy. Appropriately functional chairs that are suitable include a simple folding chair, with a seat that is flat or tilted down slightly. We do not normally recommend the backless folding yoga prop chair because it does not support the back; it is not safe for those who are unable to sit forward on the seat of the chair, for sitting back in Yoga Rest Pose (pages 180), or for meditation.

When participating in a chair-yoga class, you may not have the pleasure of choosing your chair and will have to make do with what the venue provides. Nevertheless, it is wise to look over your chair closely to maximize safety:

- See if the chair back or seat is ripped. If so, change it out for another one if possible.

- Look for loose parts. For example, check to be sure that the legs, seat, and back are stable and secure, with no loose screws or damage that might compromise safety.

- Be sure that the chair doesn't slide on the floor surface. To prevent this, place the back legs of the chair on a yoga mat or put coasters underneath the chair legs. (Recycling an old yoga mat by cutting it up is great for this.)

- If the only chairs available are office chairs that swivel, make sure the castor wheels are secure and locked.

In addition, when using chairs with arms, remember that some poses will need to be adapted further. When chair yoga becomes what one student affectionately called "armchair yoga," some postures, such as Dancer Pose, may need to be done from the front of the chair rather than from the side. Also, those on wheelchairs need to be sure that the wheels of the chair are locked for safety.

To ensure proper postural alignment, you can use props to adjust yourself on any chair, making modifications so that the chair suits you and brings ease into your practice. For more details, see the props section below (page 215) and the section on the seat of the chair and overall safety in chapter 6 (page 52).

Tips for Creating a Safe and Welcoming Space to Teach Chair Yoga

- Make sure there is enough room for each student and their chair.

- Check that all the chairs are sturdy and secure.

- Place each chair on a yoga mat or chair coasters if needed to keep from sliding.

- Make sure the chairs are spaced properly so that all students, including those in the back and on the sides, have a clear view of you and can hear you.

- Do a risk assessment of the facility or venue, checking for emergency exits, water availability, restrooms, and other health policies and safety procedures, including implementing any required local coronavirus guidelines.

- Be sure the venue is accessible to people with disabilities.

- Check that lighting and windows are appropriate for your students.

- If desired, bring in music as appropriate, such as peaceful music that promotes awareness, relaxation, and meditation, or upbeat music that invites energy. (See precaution on page 212 in case of hearing impairment.)

- An unscented or battery-operated candle is lovely.

- Please be aware of the use of essential oils or scents due to allergies. (See precaution on page 212.)

- Turn off all cell phones.

- Have a range of props available, if possible, and check that they are in good condition and suitable for how they are to be used. Encourage students to use props as needed and even bring their own if they wish. Be sure any props are placed safely—for instance, under chairs—to avoid trip hazards.

- When teaching online, remind students of the safety points above and ask them to take responsibility themselves for setting up a safe environment and practicing safely wherever they are.

- If appropriate, suggest that students wear clothing that is comfortable for moving and breathing. For safety, avoid wearing items (for example, belts) that may feel too restrictive or that might get caught on the chair.

- With everyone practicing yoga together on their own chair, you create a level-playing field so all your students feel welcome, included, and able to experience and access all the benefits of a full yoga practice.

Using Props and Assists

We love props! In yoga, a prop is generally considered to be a physical object such as a block, brick, bolster, strap, even a yoga mat that can be used to assist us in doing a pose or other yoga technique to achieve the benefits desired. Yet the use of props is only one means of providing an "assist." Below we describe a range of assists that can help enhance anyone's chair-yoga experience.

Verbal instructions: When teaching, use clear and accessible language, appropriate for your audience, to describe options and guide students with words. Remember matrika shakti!

Visual demonstrations: Show students options through body movements and visual cues that support your verbal directions. Remember levels of flexibility and start with the most basic option.

Physical assists: Props can help achieve a particular benefit—for example, using blocks or books under the foot to access a different level of flexibility in Cow Face Pose (page 96) or making a nest of soft props to increase comfort in Yoga Rest Pose (page 180). Another physical assist is touch, traditionally known as adjustments in yoga, when a yoga teacher touches a part of the student's body—often a limb—to guide movement or improve alignment. For example, for Dancer Pose, a teacher may assist a student using a wheelchair (page 103) by helping them to raise and stretch their arm to gain the benefits of this movement. For caregivers and yoga teachers, there may be local laws governing rules around physical touch for safeguarding reasons; be sure to check beforehand. In addition, always receive consent from a client or student before touching or making a physical adjustment. For any assists requiring touch by a teacher or caregiver, be sure to obtain consent beforehand in accordance with Yoga Alliance's Code of Conduct on consent-based touch.[19]

Self-assists: Students can assist themselves, and teachers can invite them to do so, through the use of props. In addition, students can add focus and strength to a practice using their own limbs—for instance, by using their hands under their thigh to lift and support their leg in Tree Pose or incorporating hand mudras into breathing, movement, and meditation practices. Students should set up their props before class begins so that they are within reach.

When choosing props, you can invest in yoga props specially designed for use with yoga postures or simply use items at hand if you're practicing at home. For instance, a cushion or rolled-up towel or yoga mat can be placed behind your torso to bring your back forward and lengthen your spine into postural alignment. A large beach towel or blanket can be rolled up, draped around your shoulders, and tucked under your armpits for meditation in Sitting Mountain or Yoga Rest Pose to keep your neck safe. If your feet don't touch the ground in Sitting Mountain or any other pose, use blocks or books to "build a floor" under your feet, raising the ground up to suit your body. For more examples of the use of props, see various poses in chapter 9. There are limitless ways to use props to make your chair-yoga practice more beneficial based on your own body and the intention(s) you set—remember to use your own sat nam and creativity to experiment and explore.

13

Building a Lakshmi Voelker Method Sequence

Yoga is the art and science of living.

—INDRA DEVI

NOW THAT YOU'VE had the opportunity to explore forty poses using our approach to chair yoga, it's time to create your own chair-yoga sequences and put together a complete practice that includes breath, movement, and meditation/relaxation. The basic outline for a Lakshmi Voelker Chair Yoga Sequence is opening, warm-ups, asanas, cool downs (rest), and closing, and the chart below provides a structure you can use to guide and inspire you, whether you're creating a practice for yourself or teaching others. Remember to bring your sat nam to the process!

First, settle in and come into the physical and mental space for practicing chair yoga (Sitting Mountain, opening). Now bring your attention to your breath, to the natural flow of your inbreath and outbreath. When you're ready, choose to alter it with a specific pranayama, if desired.

Movements include warming up your joints first to avoid injury, followed by a choice of asanas, depending on the intention of your practice. After movement, let your body-mind calm and rest through meditation or relaxation. End with something that brings the practice to a close (a mantra, reading, mudra, affirmation, pranayama) before consciously coming back into the space where your practice began.

Parts of a Lakshmi Voelker Method Sequence	Tips and Examples
Sitting Mountain	Come into postural alignment. Feel your body along with the grounding sensations of a mountain.
Opening	Set an intention for the practice. Chant a mantra. Share an affirmation.
Pranayama	Bring awareness to the importance of your breath.
Warm-ups	Use warm-ups to awaken your spine, joints, and muscles while bringing in mindfulness and honoring levels of flexibility.
Asanas	Explore various poses with breath and awareness of levels of flexibility.
Cool down	Allow your body-mind to integrate the benefits of the practice and find comfort and rest with a meditation or relaxation.
Closing	End with something that marks this practice as a special time of self-care, such as a favorite short reading, mudra, and namaste.

You can use this structure for a yoga session of any length; you can include some or all of the parts listed; and you can change the order to suit the chair-yoga session you want to practice or teach. If you're new to yoga or if you're short on time, start with something small—even one minute of yoga is still yoga.

When you are creating a sequence, you can choose practices that you are familiar with as well as new ones. Incorporating both—something familiar to support, maintain, and strengthen your body-mind and something fresh to stimulate new movements and patterns in your body-mind—can be very effective.

The Lakshmi Voelker Method Sequences

Below are some sequences you can follow using the chair-yoga poses in this book.

POSES THAT FOCUS ON BALANCE
Sitting Mountain
Extended One-Leg Pose
Tree Pose
Dancer Pose
Eagle Pose
Boat Pose
Squat Pose

POSES THAT FOCUS ON BONE STRENGTH
Sitting Mountain
Tree Pose
Chair Pose
Triangle Pose
Warrior II
Spinal Twist
Cobra Pose
Bridge Pose
Locust Pose

POSES THAT FOCUS ON MUSCLE STRENGTH
Warrior poses
Gate Pose
Downward-Facing Dog
Boat Pose
Pigeon Pose
Plank Pose
Chair Pose

POSES THAT RELAX AND RESTORE
Sitting Mountain
Bound Angle Pose
Child's Pose
Forward Fold
Knee-to-Chest Pose
Pigeon Pose
Yoga Rest Pose

WARRIOR SERIES
Sitting Mountain
Warrior I
Warrior II
Triangle Pose
Reverse Warrior
Humble Warrior
High Lunge Pose
Revolved Lunge Pose

SUN SALUTATION
Sitting Mountain
Upward Salute
Half Forward Fold
Lunge Pose
Plank Pose
Eight-Limbed Pose
Cobra Pose
Downward-Facing Dog
Lunge Pose
Half Forward Fold
Upward Salute
Sitting Mountain

MOON SALUTATION
Sitting Mountain
Crescent Moon Pose
Victory Pose
Five-Pointed Star Pose
Triangle Pose
Revolved Lunge Pose
Squat Pose
Revolved Lunge Pose
Triangle Pose
Five-Pointed Star Pose
Victory Pose
Crescent Moon Pose
Sitting Mountain

POSES "AT YOUR DESK" AT HOME OR IN THE OFFICE
Sitting Mountain—
    to improve posture
Tree Pose—for a flexible spine
Eagle Pose—for healthy joints
Squat Pose—
    to relax your lower back
Knee-to-Chest Pose—to
    support good digestion
Spinal Twist—to release tension
    in your spine

Glossary

Adi Mudra: "First" hand gesture.

Affirmation: A positive statement that one seeks to remember and absorb.

Ajna chakra: "Brow" or "Third Eye" chakra located between the eyes.

Alignment: The proper positioning of parts of the body.

Alternate Nostril Breathing: Subtle energy-cleansing breathing technique.

Anahata chakra: "Heart" chakra located at the chest.

Anjali Mudra: "Divine offering" hand gesture.

Anuloma Viloma pranayama: Alternate Nostril Breathing. *Anuloma* can be translated as "with the grain" and *viloma* as "against the grain," indicating the balancing qualities of alternating movement between the left and right nostrils.

Asana: "Seat." Third limb in Patanjali's Ashtanga (eight-limb) yoga path. Refers to body posture, pose, or position.

Ashtanga: "Eight limbs" of yoga. Refers to Patanjali's classification of classical yoga. Also the name of a dynamic, flowing yoga style.

Beginner's mind: Having an attitude of openness, eagerness, and lack of preconceptions when studying a subject.

Bhramari pranayama: "Humming bee" breathing technique.

Bija mantra: "Seed" mantra. One-syllable sound or word repeated in the form of a chant.

Breathing technique: A method of focusing on inhalation and exhalation.

Chakra: "Wheel" or "circle." Yoga system of seven energy points in the body.

Chant: A repeated rhythmic syllable, word, or phrase.

Chin Mudra: "Consciousness" hand gesture.

Coherent breathing: Long, slow breathing at the rate of five or six breaths per minute with no pauses.

Cooling breath : A breath that cools the body, adds moisture to the system, and soothes anger. See Sitali pranayama and Sitkari pranayama.

Dharana: "Concentration." Sixth limb in Patanjali's Ashtanga (eight-limb) yoga path. Refers to mastery of attention and intention.

Dhyana: "Meditation." Seventh limb in Patanjali's Ashtanga (eight-limb) yoga path. Refers to witness awareness.

Dirgha: "Long." Three-part calming, grounding, and focusing breath that encourages spaciousness in the lungs.

Drishti: "Gaze" or "view." Refers to the focus of the eyes.

Eight limbs of yoga: Patanjali's classification of classical yoga.

Hakini Mudra: "Power" hand gesture.

Hamsa: "I am that." Also known as the "mantra of the self" or "my own mantra."

Hatha yoga: Refers to yoga focusing on postures and body movement. *Hatha* means "force," and the two syllables separately mean "sun" (*ha*) and "moon" (*tha*).

Intention: Statement of purpose or aim to achieve something, representing a commitment to act in the present moment.

Japamala: String of beads used for meditation, traditionally composed of 108 (+1) beads. *Japa* means "repetition" and *mala* means "garland."

Jnana Mudra: "Knowledge" or "wisdom" hand gesture.

Kripalu: "Compassionate." Refers to the largest yoga center based in North America as well as the style of yoga taught there. Key principle of the Lakshmi Voelker Method.

Lakshmi: "Abundance." Lakshmi is the Hindu goddess of prosperity. Key principle of the Lakshmi Voelker Method.

Levels of flexibility: Range of motion used in the Lakshmi Voelker Method to offer safe, effective, inclusive options for any yoga technique that honor where each person is in the present moment.

Manipura chakra: "Navel" chakra located at the abdomen.

Mantra: "Instrument of thought." Repeated sounds or words chanted in a songlike fashion, either spoken aloud or repeated silently.

Matrika shakti: "Power of the word." Key principle of the Lakshmi Voelker Method.

Metta: "Loving-kindness." A form of Buddhist meditation that fosters positive energy and kindness toward ourselves and others.

Mindfulness: A mental state achieved by focusing one's awareness on the present moment.

Mudra: "Gesture" or "seal." Refers to the symbolic or ritual holding of a part of the body, most often the hands and fingers, in a particular position.

Muladhara chakra: "Root" chakra located at the base of the spine.

Nadi Shodhana pranayama: Alternate Nostril Breathing. Sanskrit name can be translated as "channel cleaning" or "cleansing the energy pathways," indicating physical and spiritual clearing of the nostrils.

Namaste: "I honor the light within you that resides in me." A traditional and respectful Indian greeting that translates literally as "I bow to you."

Niyama: "Observance." Second limb in Patanjali's Ashtanga (eight-limb) yoga path. Refers to five guidelines for personal behavior. Key principle of the Lakshmi Voelker Method.

OM: A well-known mantra and sacred symbol of many traditions and religions. Often referred to as "the universal sound."

Padma Mudra: "Lotus" flower hand gesture.

Patanjali: Great sage of yoga philosophy known for his classic work, *The Yoga Sutras.*

Pranayama: "Extension of life-giving force." Fourth limb in Patanjali's Ashtanga (eight-limb) yoga path. Refers to the practice of breath control.

Pratyahara: "Withdrawal of the senses." Fifth limb in Patanjali's Ashtanga (eight-limb) yoga path. Refers to closing off external distractions to turn the mind inward.

Pratipaksha bhavana: "Cultivating opposites." Yogic practice of shifting negative ways of thinking. Key principle of the Lakshmi Voelker Method.

Sahasrara chakra: "Crown" chakra located at the top of the head.

Samadhi: "Intense self-absorption." Eighth limb in Patanjali's Ashtanga (eight-limb) yoga path. Refers to a state of being settled in pure, unbounded awareness.

Sanskrit: An ancient language of India and the original language of yoga.

Sat-chit-ananda: "Create-Sustain-Dissolve." *Sat* means "truth" or "existence," *chit* means "consciousness," and *ananda* means "bliss." Key principle of the Lakshmi Voelker Method.

Sat nam: "True identity" or "true self." The two syllables separately mean "true" or "everlasting" (*sat*) and "name" (*nam*). Key principle of the Lakshmi Voelker Method.

Shaktipat: "Transmission of wisdom," or literally "prostration of strength." Key principle of the Lakshmi Voelker Method.

Shanti: "Peace."

Siddha Yoga: Yoga tradition that focuses on the path of self-realization.

Sitali pranayama: Breathing technique where the breath is drawn through the rolled-up tongue to cool and moisturize the body.

Sitkari pranayama: Breathing technique where the breath is drawn in over the surface of the tongue to cool and moisturize the body.

Sutra: "Thread." Aphorism in Sanskrit literature.

Svadhishthana chakra: "Sacral" chakra located just below the navel.

Ujjayi pranayama: "Victorious" breath. A warming breath with sound from the throat like ocean waves.

Vishuddha chakra: "Throat" chakra located at the throat.

Yama: "Restraint." First limb in Patanjali's Ashtanga (eight-limb) yoga path. Refers to five guidelines for social behavior. Key principle of the Lakshmi Voelker Method.

Yoga: "Union" or integration of body, mind, and spirit.

Yoga Nidra: "Yogic sleep." Guided meditation featuring rotation of consciousness for deep relaxation.

Notes

1. Printed with kind permission from the author.

2. Achraf Ammar et al., "Effects of COVID-19 Home Confinement on Eating Behaviour and Physical Activity: Results of the ECLB-COVID19 International Online Survey," *Nutrients* 12, no. 6 (2020): 1583.

3. Audrius Kulikajevas, Rytis Maskeliunas, and Robertus Damaševičius, "Detection of Sitting Posture Using Hierarchical Image Composition and Deep Learning," *PeerJ Computer Science* 7 (2021): e442.

4. Sophie Carter et al., "Regular Walking Breaks Prevent the Decline in Cerebral Blood Flow Associated with Prolonged Sitting," *Journal of Applied Physiology* 125, no. 3 (2018): 790–98.

5. Megan Teychenne, Sarah A. Costigan, and Kate Parker, "The Association between Sedentary Behavior and Risk of Anxiety: A Systematic Review," *BMC Public Health* 15, no. 1 (2015): 513; Gabriel Zieff et al., "Targeting Sedentary Behavior as a Feasible Health Strategy During COVID-19," *Translational Behavioral Medicine* 11, no. 3 (2021): 826–31.

6. World Health Organization, *WHO Guidelines on Physical Activity and Sedentary Behaviour* (Geneva: World Health Organization, 2020).

7. Commentary by T. Krishnamacharya, *Yoga Sutras* 1:34, https://yogastudies.org/sutra/yoga-sutra chapter-1-verse-34/.

8. Printed with kind permission from Kripalu School of Yoga.

9. Kripalu's press-point system was developed by Shankari Michelle Deschamps and Christopher Baxter. Special thanks to Michelle Dalbec and Rudy Peirce for sharing this information with Lakshmi and Lakshmi Voelker Chair Yoga.

10. Richard P. Brown, Patricia L. Gerbarg, and Fred Meunch, "Breathing Practices for Treatment of Psychiatric and Stress-Related Medical Conditions," *Psychiatric Clinics of North America* 36 (2013): 121–40.

11. For further details on consent-based touch, see Yoga Alliance's Code of Conduct, available on the Yoga Alliance website. See: "Code of Conduct," https://www.yogaalliance.org/aboutya/ourpolicies/codeofconduct.

12. Mayo Clinic, "Exercise: When to check with your doctor first," February 24, 2021, https://www.mayoclinic .org/healthy-lifestyle/fitness/in-depth/exercise/art-20047414.

13. Herbert Benson, *The Relaxation Response* (New York: William Morrow, 1975).

14. American professor Jon Kabat-Zinn described mindfulness as "the awareness that emerges through paying attention on purpose, in the present moment, and nonjudgmentally to the unfolding of experience moment by moment." In the 1970s, Kabat-Zinn recruited chronically ill patients who did not respond well to Western-based medical treatments to a program of intensive training in mindfulness meditation; his eight-week Mindfulness-Based Stress Reduction (MBSR) course delivered positive results in relieving stress, pain, and illness. Since then, research on mindfulness has proliferated and many treatment models have been developed. For more on the research of Jon Kabat-Zinn, see Kabat-Zinn, "Mindfulness-Based Interventions in Context: Past, Present, and Future," *Clinical Psychology Science Practice* 10 (2003): 144–56. For more on recent research on mindfulness-based treatment models, see D. Zhang, E. K. P. Lee, E. C. W. Mak, C. Y. Ho, and S. Y. S. Wong, "Mindfulness-Based Interventions: An Overall Review," *British Medical Journal* 138, no. 1 (2021): 41–57.

15. Adapted with kind permission from Heather Mason, The Minded Institute, London.

16. Adapted with kind permission from Stephanie Shanti Bosanko.

17. Adapted with kind permission from Heather Mason, The Minded Institute, London.

18. See J. H. Lee, The Effects of Music on Pain: A Meta-Analysis," *Journal of Music Therapy* 53, no. 4 (2016): 430–77. Erratum in: *Journal of Music Therapy* 58, no. 3 (2021): 372. N. Daykin, L. Mansfield, C. Meads, et al., "What Works for Wellbeing? A Systematic Review of Wellbeing Outcomes for Music and Singing in Adults," *Perspectives in Public Health* 138, no. 1 (2018): 39–46.

19. For more details on consent-based touch, see Yoga Alliance's Code of Conduct, available on the Yoga Alliance website. See: "Code of Conduct," https://www.yogaalliance.org/aboutya/ourpolicies /codeofconduct.

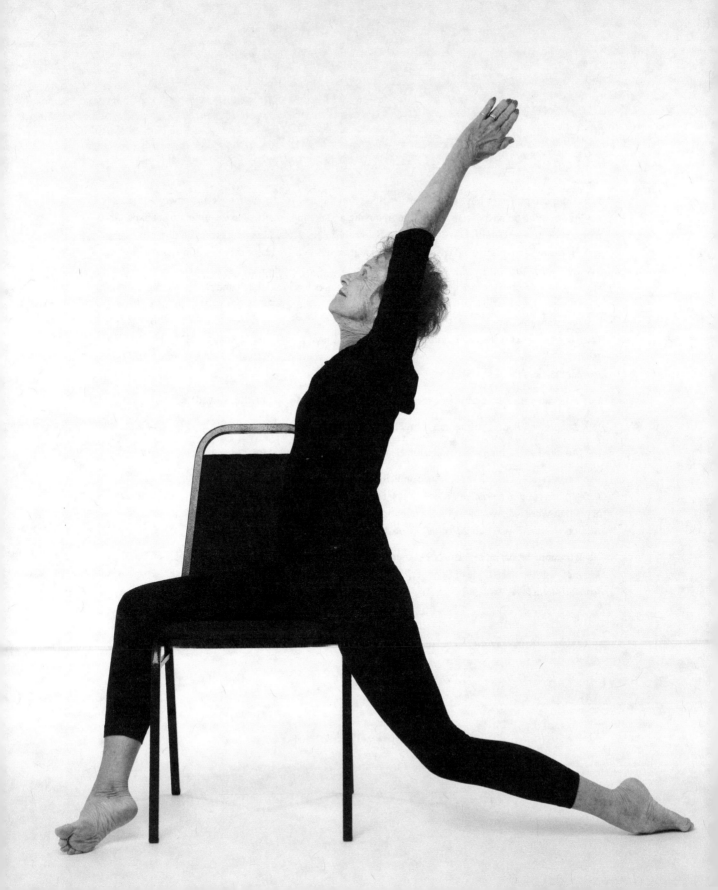

Index of Poses

Pose		Sanskrit	Pages
1	Boat Pose	Navasana	84–85
2	Bound Angle Pose	Baddha Konasana	86–87
3	Bridge Pose	Setu Bandha Sarvangasana/ Setu Bandhasana	88–89
4	Chair Pose	Utkatasana	90–91
5	Child's Pose	Balasana	92–93
6	Cobra Pose	Bhujangasana	94–95
7	Cow Face Pose	Gomukhasana	96–97
8	Crescent Moon Pose	Indudalasana	98–99
9	Dancer Pose	Natarajasana	100–103
10	Downward-Facing Dog	Adho Mukha Shvanasana	104–5
11	Eagle Pose	Garudasana	106–7
12	Eight-Limbed Pose	Ashtanga Namaskara	108–9
13	Extended One-Leg Pose	Utthita Eka Padasana	110–11
14	Fish Pose	Matsyasana	112–13
15	Five-Pointed Star Pose	Utthita Tadasana	114–15

About the Authors

LAKSHMI VOELKER, C-IAYT, E-RYT 500, created Lakshmi Voelker Chair Yoga™ in 1982 when one of her students was stricken with arthritis and could no longer get down on and up from the floor to practice yoga. Since then, Lakshmi's innovative approach to adaptive yoga has inspired thousands of people to practice chair yoga. She lives with her husband and pets in Huntington Beach, California.

Lakshmi has more than fifty years of experience in the yoga and fitness industry, specializing in office, senior, and adaptive fitness. She has certified more than 2,500 chair-yoga teachers nationally and internationally in the Lakshmi Voelker Method, including health-care professionals at the Mayo Clinic, the New York City Department of Education, and the Veterans Health Administration. She regularly runs trainings at Kripalu Center for Yoga and Health and offers online teacher trainings worldwide.

Trained at Kripalu and in the Siddha Yoga tradition, Lakshmi has studied, practiced, and taught yoga and other Eastern disciplines since 1969. From her early years, she integrated these disciplines with Western health concepts. Her focus has always been to improve her students' health and wellness by making yoga accessible to the broadest audience possible. Combining intuition, humor, and compassion, Lakshmi guides and mentors her students and teachers, enthusing them to build special connections in their own communities through chair yoga.

LIZ OPPEDIJK, BCYT, E-RYT 500, MSc, came to yoga in her fifties following serious illness and injury. Through yoga, her recovery became a transformation, inspiring her to establish Accessible Chair Yoga CIC, a nonprofit social enterprise. Her aim is to bring chair yoga to every nursing home in the UK and beyond. She resides in St. Albans, England, with her two grown children living close by in London.

Liz is a leading expert on chair yoga in the UK and has completed several research projects into the health and social benefits of yoga. She trains chair-yoga teachers to bring yoga to those with accessibility needs, including and enthusing those who have never considered yoga to be for them. She lectures, writes, and facilitates trainings on chair and accessible yoga, Parkinson's disease, and dementia, reaching audiences both in the UK and abroad.

Initially Liz trained in vinyasa and hot yoga before discovering chair yoga with Lakshmi Voelker. She went on to train as a yoga therapist with the Minded Institute in London, bringing both a holistic and specialist approach to yoga on the chair. At the heart of her work—mentoring, teacher training, teaching—is the drive to empower others. Her students describe her as thoughtful and practical, knowledgeable and inspiring. Liz aspires for chair yoga to be practiced with authenticity and joy.